THE S FACTOR DIET

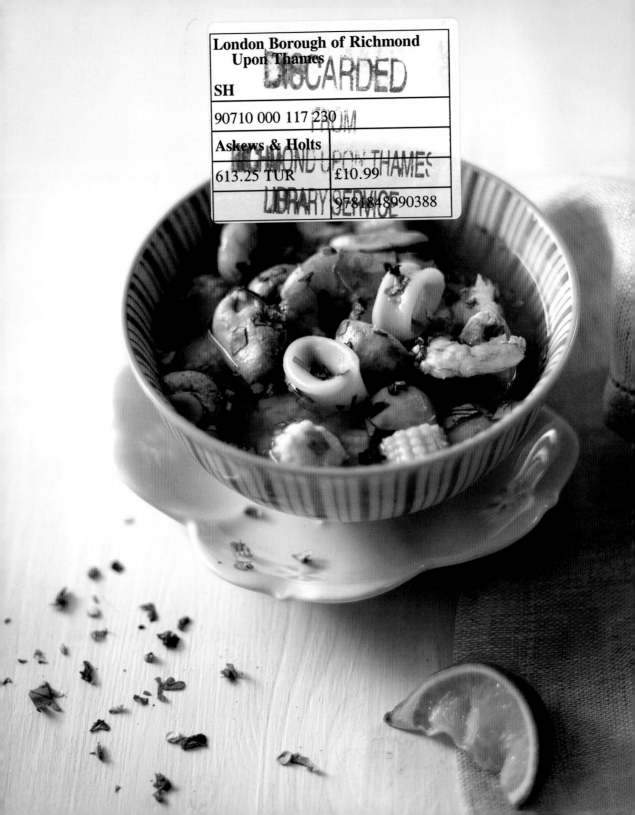

THE S FACTOR DIET

The Happiest Way to Lose Weight

LOWRI TURNER

DUNCAN BAIRD PUBLISHERS

LONDON

The S Factor Diet

Lowri Turner

First published in the United Kingdom and Ireland
in 2013 by
Duncan Baird Publishers Ltd
Sixth Floor, Castle House
75–76 Wells Street
London W1T 3QH

Conceived, created and designed by
Duncan Baird Publishers

Managing Editor: Grace Cheetham
Editor: Krissy Mallett
Managing Designer: Manisha Patel
Designer: Gail Jones
Production: Uzma Taj
Commissioned Photography: Toby Scott
Food Stylist: Jayne Cross
Prop Stylist: Lucy Harvey

British Library Cataloguing-in-Publication Data:
A CIP record for this book is available from the
British Library

ISBN: 978-1-84899-038-8

10 9 8 7 6 5 4 3 2 1

For my children, Griffin, Merlin and Ariel

Typeset in Frutiger
Colour reproduction by XY Digital UK
Printed in Singapore by Imago

Publisher's note
While every care has been taken in compiling the recipes for this
book, Duncan Baird Publishers, or any other persons who have
been involved in working on this publication, cannot accept
responsibility for any errors or omissions, inadvertent or not, that
may be found in the recipes or text, nor for any problems that
may arise as a result of preparing one of these recipes. If you are
pregnant or breastfeeding or have any special dietary requirements
or medical conditions, it is advisable to consult a medical
professional before following any of the recipes contained in this
book. If you are clinically depressed, diet alone won't make you
happy – seek medical attention.

Notes on the recipes
Unless otherwise stated:
Use medium fruit and vegetables
Use fresh ingredients, including herbs and chillies
Do not mix metric and imperial measurements
1 tsp = 5ml 1 tbsp = 15ml 1 cup = 250ml

Author's acknowledgments
Many thanks to my children, Griffin, Merlin and Ariel, for tasting
some of the recipes, admittedly with some degree of suspicion
(Merlin: "Does it have vegetables in it?"), as well as for just being
a constant source of interest and fun. Also thanks to Toby, Gail,
Jayne and Lucy for making the recipes look so good, and to Grace
and Krissy for their advice and editing flair.

Note to the reader
Hormones and neurotransmitters are both types of chemical
messengers which activate systems in our body such as fat burning
and fat storage. Hormones are released by endocrine glands, while
neurotransmitters are released by nerves. The leptin hormone and
adrenal hormones such as cortisol and adrenaline, can impact on
our weight, as can the neurotransmitters serotonin and dopamine
– you will read about all of them in this book. For simplicity, I
have used the term "S Factor hormones" to refer to this group of
hormones and neurotransmitters.

Contents

Introduction

So what do I know about diets? Well, I used to go on a lot of them. I also used to fall off a lot of them. Throughout my teens, twenties and early thirties my life was divided into three categories: on a diet, falling off a diet and eating everything in sight because I was about to go on a diet.

What made it worse was that people treated me differently according to how fat I was. When I was slim, men liked me, chatted me up and asked me out. When I was fat, either I was invisible, or teenage boys made rude comments in the street. The flipside was that as a skinny minnie, women were deeply suspicious. Only when I regained the weight did I get to rejoin the sisterhood.

But hang on, aren't we the same people however much padding we have? The world doesn't seem to think so.

Most diet books appear to have been written by people who have never been fat. They say that looks don't matter. I spent so many years being fat, thin and anywhere in between, I can say that looks do matter – to you and to everyone else who feels they have a right to an opinion. I can still vividly remember the embarrassment of sitting on a tube train as a teen and trying to prevent the side of my size 18 legs touching the person next to me. What I wanted to know back then was if other people could eat normally and stay the same size, why couldn't I?

Fast-forward a few years (and three babies later) and I am now a stable size 10. No more keeping black trousers in three sizes; no more beginning every day vowing to stick to a diet before buckling at 6pm and eating an entire tray of Mars Bar ice creams; and no more feeling guilty, angry and depressed about food.

I won't claim to be a food saint. I have my "off" days, but I don't obsess about it any more. I feel happy and healthy. I watch what I eat because I know what my personal potholes are. I feed my brain and my body the right food because I know how much better I feel when I do. I will also admit to a large dose of vanity – I want to be able to fit into my clothes.

So, what's changed? They say knowledge is a powerful thing and for me, it has been a revelation. When I was trying to get pregnant for the first time 13 years ago, I was diagnosed with polycystic ovarian syndrome (PCOS). PCOS is a blood sugar disorder that can cause excessive weight gain. I wasn't given any advice, only fertility drugs that made me inflate like the Michelin Man. This was disastrous when I was a TV presenter and had to have a camera pointed at me from unflattering angles. However, it was the first part of the puzzle….

Secondly, I had a hyperactive son and doctors suggested I change his diet. I then divorced (for the first time, ahem…) and the stress made me comfort eat. I also developed rosacea – a skin condition that you can recognise by a butterfly shaped redness across your nose and cheeks. I bought loads of creams but nothing helped. The clues were there – change what you eat, Lowri.

Still, I didn't really want to become a health freak. I thought those people were boring, and besides, as a working single mum I was too busy and exhausted. My job was to go on TV and be cheerful and THIN. I was propping myself up on nicotine, caffeine and sugar, but my body was burning out, even if I was ignoring it.

My rock bottom finally came when I developed a rash on the inside of my hands that was so bad I couldn't drive. The doctor put me on hydrocortisone, but also asked me if I had an allergy to dairy foods. I thought back to a year before when another doctor had suggested that a combination of stress and eating a lot of ice cream might be a contributing factor to my rosacea. The bottom line was that my diet was making me ill.

So I started to research how food could make me look and feel better. As I changed my eating habits, my weight began to stabilize and I felt more energetic and positive. Most importantly, I began to feel in control of my eating. To those who have never had an issue with food this may seem minor. However, for someone who would start with one biscuit, then finish the packet and throw away the wrapper to hide the evidence, it was the "Eureka!" moment. Gone was the girl who chain-smoked and had a fridge under her desk full of champagne and drawer in her desk permanently stocked with chocolate. I was now a health food convert.

In 2005, I began to study nutrition with a view to changing my career. To be honest, I thought it would be pretty easy. Instead, there was a solid year of studying the science of anatomy and physiology. The more I learnt, the more I began to understand why so many of us struggle with food. I learnt how unstable blood sugar levels lead to unstable moods and this in turn leads to cravings, bingeing and weight gain. Still, with my history of weight warfare, I of all people know that most of us find it hard to stick to diets.

I opened the doors to my first weight loss clients in 2009 and it was all going swimmingly. OK, there was the occasional client who didn't seem to be able to stick to their diet but I told myself that "8 out of 10 ain't bad". Still, it got me thinking. I did a bit more research and started experimenting (in a nice way) with my clients. I soon realized I had missed something blindingly obvious: overeating is a form of self-medication and not just in a metaphorical sense.

I now believe that overeating can be a physiological attempt to correct imbalances in what I call the S Factor hormones – natural chemicals we are all supposed to produce in abundance, but which some of us don't. Scientists now know that certain foods stimulate the production of particular hormones (leptin and adrenal hormones such as cortisol) and neurotransmitters (serotonin and dopamine). These S Factor hormones control how hungry you feel and how satisfied you are after eating. Craving unhealthy foods is the body's ill-advised attempt to boost these hormones and control blood sugar levels. So by designing my diets I was trying to persuade clients to eat salad when their brains were screaming "CHOCOLATE!" I was suggesting they might enjoy an apple when their brains were bellowing, "I WANT A BIG BOWL OF PASTA NOW!" Frankly, it's a wonder they didn't throttle me.

From a lot of complicated science, my simple message is this: you can lose weight if you get your S Factor hormones working properly.

How do you do that? Well, that's what this book is all about. Fill in a series of questionnaires to establish your unique needs. Then you can customize a food plan of delicious meals to suit you. And, I haven't just pulled this stuff out of thin air – I've perfected the S Factor diet after working with real weight loss clients. I know it works and I know it can work for you. Read on and learn the science behind the diet.

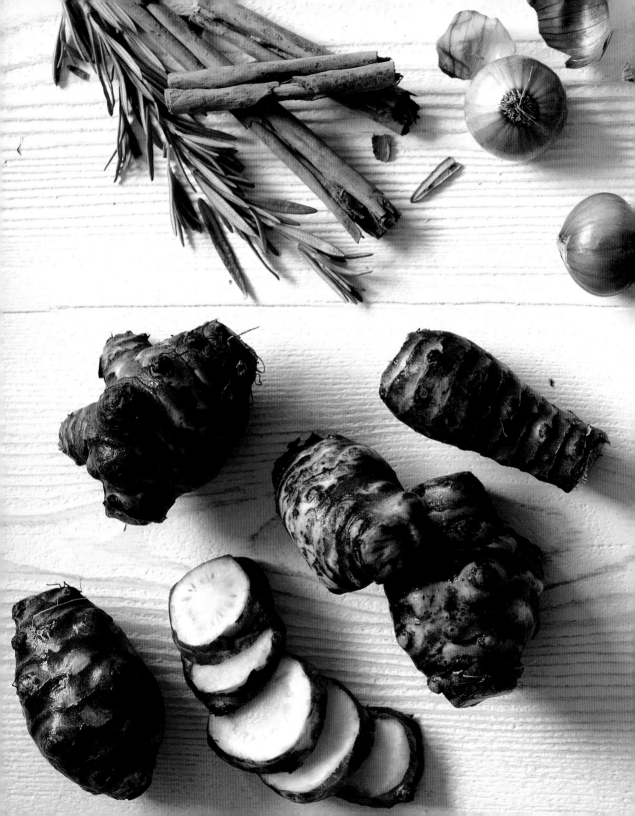

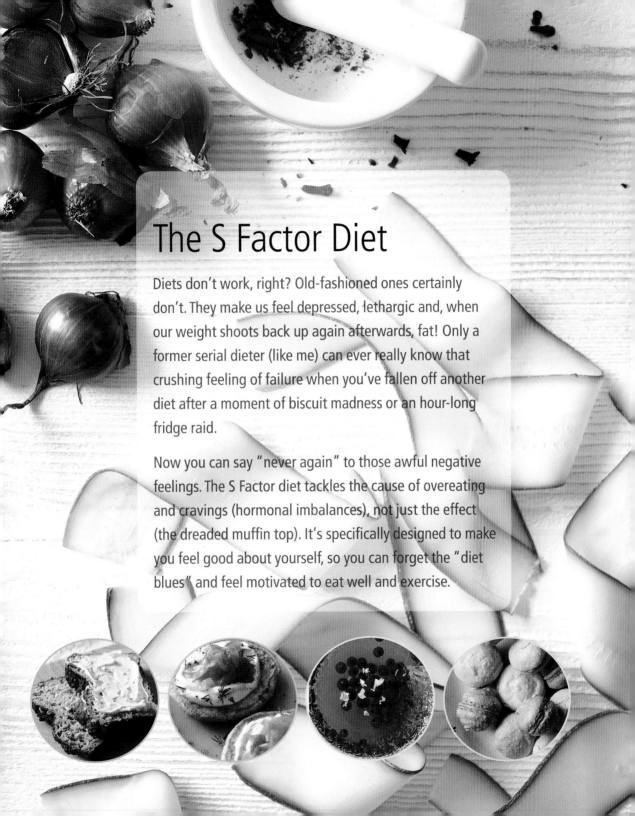

The S Factor Diet

Diets don't work, right? Old-fashioned ones certainly don't. They make us feel depressed, lethargic and, when our weight shoots back up again afterwards, fat! Only a former serial dieter (like me) can ever really know that crushing feeling of failure when you've fallen off another diet after a moment of biscuit madness or an hour-long fridge raid.

Now you can say "never again" to those awful negative feelings. The S Factor diet tackles the cause of overeating and cravings (hormonal imbalances), not just the effect (the dreaded muffin top). It's specifically designed to make you feel good about yourself, so you can forget the "diet blues" and feel motivated to eat well and exercise.

The S Factor Diet

Scientists now know that certain foods have a direct effect on the way we think and feel. The S Factor diet goes one step further. It is a diet designed to lift your mood, reduce your appetite and burn fat. Let's start with a few questions:

- Do you want to lose weight?
- Do you have a wardrobe full of clothes you can't fit into?
- Are you an emotional or comfort eater?
- Do you start diets and fall off them?
- Do you have a gym membership you never use?
- Do you crave chocolate, pasta or ice cream (especially at night)?
- Do you go out shopping for clothes, go into the changing room and when nothing fits end up buying a pair of shoes, handbag or a lipstick instead?

If you answered "yes" to any of the above questions, the S Factor diet is for you. It's been designed to help you lose weight by getting all your S Factor hormones working properly. These natural chemicals control how hungry you feel and how satisfied you are after eating. They can boost your mood, give you more energy and bump up your motivation. Most importantly, they can help you burn fat.

When You're Happy You Eat Less

Certainly it's possible to lose weight when you feel depressed. I was once dumped by a boyfriend in the middle of a busy high street. (He thought I wouldn't make a scene in public – how wrong he was!) Anyway, I was so devastated that I lived pretty much on Chardonnay for a month. I lost loads of weight and

people said I looked fabulous (I felt terrible). But, in the main, it's when we are happy that we eat less. We take the time to look after ourselves. When we are happy, we don't need to tranquilize ourselves with big bowls of pasta or huge slices of cake. Our appetite is reduced and our motivation to get up and do things is increased.

You Can Eat Yourself Happy

The S Factor diet is based on the scientifically proven link between certain hormones and the foods we eat. These amazing substances are produced naturally and in abundance by our own bodies. All we have to do is give our bodies the raw material to make them – just like putting petrol in a car. Once you are fuelled with the right amounts of these special hormones, you will have a reduced appetite, fewer cravings and more motivation to exercise. You may also burn fat more effectively, sleep better, your skin and hair could improve and PMS and other conditions such as PCOS and endometriosis may also be eased.

Sounds brilliant, so why haven't you heard about this before? Mainly, it's because the science is so new. The discoveries about leptin, one of the S Factor hormones I will talk about in this book, are literally being made as I write. In-depth studies on serotonin and dopamine, two other important S Factor hormones, have only really been possible since new brain imaging techniques were developed. These discoveries have shown that we all manufacture more S Factor hormones in the gut rather than in the brain. Therefore, there is a reciprocal connection between how we feel and what we eat – it's a two-way street.

The Trouble with Diets

All this makes old-fashioned diets sound, well, old-fashioned. It also explains why so many of the diets you have been on may have failed – it's the diet that failed, not you, by the way. The problem with most diets is that they make you depressed. This isn't just because you have to live on lettuce, it's also because they starve you of the raw materials needed to make S Factor hormones. Conventional diets fall into two main types:

Low-Fat Diets

Reducing saturated fat, the type you find in meat, cheese, cream and so on, can be a good thing. For instance, there appears to be a correlation between high saturated fat intake and heart problems. Reducing trans fats is also essential. Trans fats are man-made, processed fats, produced when liquid fats are turned into solid fats via a process known as hydrogenation. Trans fats are found in cheap junk foods like petrol station pies and pasties, and have been linked with cancer. But low-fat diets can be problematic.

Low-Fat Diets Can Make You Stupid

If you cut all fat out of your diet, you may lose good omega 3, 6 and 9 fats, also known as "essential" fats. You will find essential fats in oily fish like salmon as well as in nuts, seeds and olive oil. We all need these fats to make our brains, as well as our bodies, work properly. Neural networks carry essential messages back and forth. They work a bit like electrical wiring. When they malfunction, our brain's messaging slows down, affecting our ability to focus, concentrate and think clearly.

Low-Fat Diets Can Make You Fat

Not eating enough essential fats has been directly linked to depression. What do we do when we are depressed? We eat of course, only we don't binge on broccoli, instead we crave chocolate, biscuits, cake, bread… all the things that really pack on the pounds. Low-fat diets can also be quite "sugary". By that I don't mean they are full of doughnuts. Low-fat carbohydrate foods such as rice, pasta and baked potatoes have a high GI value. GI stands for glycaemic index, which is a measure of how fast carbohydrate foods break down into sugar and hit the bloodstream. High GI foods release their sugar quickly. However, if the sugar in your blood gets too high too fast, it is stored as fat. Essential fats have also been shown to slow down the rate at which your stomach empties – slowing down the speed at which sugar enters the blood. This helps to stabilize blood sugar and reduces fat storage. So in terms of weight loss, eating some of the right fats can actually prevent you from putting on weight.

Low-Fat Diets Can Give You PMS

Every cell in our bodies has a "skin" around it partly made of essential fats. These fats are liquid at room temperature – think of runny olive oil containing essential fats as opposed to solid butter which is full of saturated fat. Essential fats keep cell walls flexible, which they need to be for all your hormones, including sex hormones such as oestrogen, to work properly. If you don't have enough of these essential fats, your hormones won't function properly. This can make symptoms of PMS worse and can aggravate hormonal conditions such as endometriosis and PCOS.

The S Factor Diet

High-Protein Diets

So, are high-protein diets any better? High-protein diets are controversial, although I don't think they're as bad as low-fat diets. However, you can have too much of a good thing and eating butter, cheese and cream all day is hardly a recipe for a long and healthy life. Apart from anything else, you are likely to become constipated and feel terrible.

High-Protein Diets Can Make You Cranky

In terms of feeling happy, high-protein diets are awful. One of the most important S Factor hormones (and the one this book is named after) is serotonin. Good serotonin levels help us feel happy.

Serotonin is made of tryptophan – an amino acid we take into our body in the form of protein. But, and it is a huge but, you need a hit of insulin for serotonin to enter the brain. How do you raise insulin? By eating sugar. High-protein diets make you depressed by cutting out the vital sugar hit you need to produce serotonin.

There are other concerns about super high-protein diets including reduced levels of vitamin C, hair loss and strain on the kidneys. However, I think their depressive effect is particularly problematic for permanent weight loss. Even body builders, who go through a protein-only "cutting" phase in the run-up to a competition, often have "cheat meals". They know that some carbohydrate is essential to give them energy to work out. It also prevents them from strangling themselves with their own teeny pants as a result of low-carb blues. The bottom line? You need to feel happy to stay slim and that's exactly what the S Factor diet helps you to do.

If happiness is a route to slimness, how do you become happy? We can't all win the lottery or bump into George Clooney in a rare girlfriend-less moment when he's decided what he really needs is a slightly dumpy, non-Hollywood partner – "Pick me, George, pick me!" Of course there are external factors that affect our happiness such as money, relationships and health, but these may be out of our control.

The S Factor Diet Makes You Happy

There is another, internal source of happiness that can help you lose weight. I'm not talking about building your self-esteem using naff affirmations of the "every day, in every way, I'm getting better and better" variety. I'm talking about taking the pragmatic approach. The S Factor diet is about changing the biochemistry of your body, and of your brain in particular, by changing the food you eat so you feel happier and healthier.

On the S Factor diet, you won't be carb-free but you will probably be eating more lean protein than you are used to. I see so many clients who think they have a healthy diet, but eat porridge for breakfast, a sandwich for lunch and pasta for dinner. They're overweight and depressed. The S Factor diet is also designed to be naturally low in saturated fats and high in hormone-friendly essential fats. The recipes are good for your heart, brain and waistline and you'll be able to satisfy your sweet tooth – another reason to feel happy.

To manufacture S Factor hormones so you can lose weight, you need to eat protein. High-protein foods like lean meat, fish, eggs and vegetable protein are at the core of the S Factor diet.

So, How Does the S Factor Diet Work?

The S Factor diet is not a crash diet that you complete and then go back to "normal" (regaining all the weight you've lost and a bit more). It is an approach to eating that can and should be maintained for life. I know that may sound slightly horrifying, but once you've got the knack of your S Factor plan, you'll look and feel so much better that you'll never want to go back.

The diet initially centres around four 14-day hormone-balancing meal plans – one for each of the S Factor hormones (see pages 32–39). Each plan is split into two phases and there are recipes for each phase. Phase 1 is the fast fat-loss stage, while Phase 2 focuses on steadier weight loss. Having two phases is also good psychologically. Your motivation is always highest at the start of any new project, be it a flat-pack or a diet, so Phase 1 is where you really attack the weight loss by sticking to around 1000–1200 calories per day. On Phase 2, your calorie count will range between 1000–1600 per day and you'll be able to enjoy a wider variety of dishes.

The meal plans are designed to help you make more of your natural appetite-suppressing, motivation-raising S Factor hormones, so you can feel happier and lose weight. But you have unique needs, and the more tailored a meal plan can be to you, the more successful you will be. This is where the questionnaires come in (see pages 20–23). Each one is designed to establish if you are just generally low in all your S Factor hormones, or if you have a particular issue with one or two of them. Once you have filled in the questionnaires, you will know which of the four 14-day meal plans is right for you.

Whichever plan you follow, you could drop up to a dress size in two weeks, but if you have more than a dress size to lose, you can stay on Phase 2 until you reach your target. And I'm not going to abandon you at that crucial point either. (Remember I used to be really good at losing weight and really rubbish at keeping it off.) Once you've reached your goal weight you can progress to one of the S Factor Lifetime Plans (see pages 124–125). Here you'll find even more recipe ideas (including more healthy carbs, like brown rice and oats). You should also allow yourself a higher calorie count of around 1500–2500 calories per day.

The S Factor Principles

The key to keeping the weight off is to stick to the principles of the S Factor diet. Look after your S Factor hormones and your weight will look after itself.

1 Eat plenty of lean protein, especially at breakfast, so you can make plenty of S Factor hormones.

2 Balance your blood sugar to keep your S Factor hormones working properly and prevent cravings. Eat low GI grains like oats and rye and pulses such as lentils and chickpeas and watch your portion sizes.

3 Include plenty of good essential fats in your diet so your brain uses your S Factor hormones properly – eat nuts, seeds and oily fish like salmon and mackerel.

4 Have your S Factor night-time snack to prevent bingeing before bedtime.

So, are you ready to get going? First here's a bit more background information. Remember: knowledge is power.

The Science Bit

OK, now pay attention and no slouching at the back. I was not a big fan of chemistry at school, but the science of weight loss, now, that's a lot more interesting, isn't it?

If you have had a long battle with food, it is too easy to dismiss this lack of self-control as you being either weak-willed or crazy. I want you to understand that it is your physiology that has been driving this behaviour so that a) you can forgive yourself, and b) you can regain control over your eating. When you can do both, you will be able to lose weight and keep it off.

All together now, "Je ne regrette rien." Well, after two divorces I have quite a lot of, if not quite regrets, things I would quite like to sweep under a very large carpet. But, that's another story and another book. This one's about shrinking those thighs.

The S Factor Hormones

So what are these natural chemicals I like to call the "S Factor hormones" and how can they help you lose weight?

There are many hormones and neurotransmitters that impact on our weight. Some are produced by glands in our bodies, some by fat cells, some in the lining of the gut and some by chewing or stretching the stomach. Scientists are discovering new ones all the time. Each one promises to be the answer to weight loss. However, the truth is that hormones work together in complex ratios and rhythms. If one becomes depleted or dominant, it affects the others. This can cause weight gain.

This is why the S Factor diet is primarily a diet that balances hormones. The aim is to get all your S Factor hormones working well so they support each other and help you to lose weight.

....

This S Factor diet focuses on four key hormones because they have the greatest effect on mood, appetite and weight. They are:

S **Serotonin: The "Good-Mood" Hormone**
Good levels of serotonin make us feel calm, contented and cravings-free. Low serotonin affects sleep, makes us feel depressed and turns us into chocoholics.

D **Dopamine: The "High-Motivation" Hormone**
Dopamine is a chemical released in our brains in response to a reward or treat. Low dopamine weakens our resolve when the office feeder proffers cupcakes, and makes walking past the chocolate display in the petrol station a nightmare.

L **Leptin: The "I'm-Not-Hungry" Hormone**
Leptin tells our brain when we have enough body fat and then reduces our appetite and speeds up our metabolism to burn off any excess. That's what it's supposed to do, but as you become overweight, it stops working properly, so you feel fat and hungry.

A **Adrenals: The "Stress" Hormones**
This group of hormones, including adrenaline and cortisol, is pumped out by the adrenal glands. The right amount of adrenal hormones gives us energy. Too much and we become tired, wired fridge-raiders.

Born to Love Cake?

Genetic factors can also play a role in weight gain. Scientists have recently focused on the so-called "Thrifty Gene Syndrome". This gives those with certain DNA the ability to store more of their food as fat – great in a famine, pretty annoying when you have an American-sized fridge and skinny jeans you want to fit into.

There has also been scientific interest in a gene that appears to code for a lower number of DRD2 dopamine receptors in the brain. It has been called the low DRD2 or low D2 gene, and is being interpreted as an "addiction gene". The thinking is, if you have fewer dopamine receptors you may try to over-stimulate the ones you do have and develop compulsive cravings.

This gene may explain why addiction seems to run in families. There certainly appears to be a correlation between this faulty gene and drinking too much. Alcohol is a sugar, so there is a certain logic in suggesting that the same gene may also lead to sugar "addiction".

It seems people who have the low DRD2 gene are vulnerable to anything that can stimulate feelings of pleasure. It could be cigarettes, a glass of wine or a slice of cake. The additional problem is that the more you stimulate the dopamine pathway in the brain, the more it needs to be stimulated – so you end up eating bigger and bigger portions of cake to get the "normal" pleasurable effect.

I always ask new clients if there is any history of compulsive behaviour (addictions to alcohol, drugs or gambling) in their family, just as I ask whether there is history of diabetes or heart disease. Indeed, a high proportion of my clients are the children of alcoholics, have had a brush with heavy drinking themselves or used club drugs as a teenager.

But the point is, you are more than your family history, more than just DNA. Many people are born into challenging backgrounds and don't develop addictions or cave in to compulsive behaviours.

Personally, I really like compulsive people – they have amazing determination and drive. Admittedly, this can propel them to do things that are fantastically unhealthy, but it can also result in high achievement. Was Sir Edmund Hillary slightly compulsive about reaching the top of Everest? Definitely. I'm not saying that all high achievers are compulsive, but it certainly helps.

Many of my clients wish they weren't compulsive, but this ambition is part of a general self-hatred that fuels over eating. When you feel bad about yourself, you don't invest in your own health. When you embrace your character and find the positives in it, even feel proud of it, you are much more likely to take care of yourself by exercising and eating well. So, give yourself a pat on the back for being compulsive, or describe yourself as "passionate" instead. Think of the things you have achieved: work projects completed, children raised, houses renovated, qualifications secured. Well done you!

If you have inherited a compulsive streak, there is more good news. Scientists now believe you can switch genes on and off and turn down the volume of your cravings with so-called "lifestyle factors", such as eating properly and exercising. The S Factor diet is designed to help you switch off your DNA-driven urge to overeat fatty and sugary foods by balancing your S Factor hormones.

Serotonin

The "Good-Mood" Hormone

Serotonin is a neurotransmitter we all make in our brains. It helps us feel happy, contented and calm. Sounds fantastic but here's the real kicker – some of us make more of it than others.

The really bad news, if you have no Y chromosome, is that women make less serotonin than men. You could argue this means we were born to be grumpy. Sorry, guys. And it gets worse. We make even less serotonin in the run up to our periods – cue PMS rage.

The reason for this is that serotonin and oestrogen are linked. When oestrogen drops in the run up to your period, so does serotonin. Chemists among you will spot another potential problem: menopause, or actually peri-menopause. This can start from about age 35 onwards, when our bodies get ready for menopause and our oestrogen production begins to slide. I see quite a few clients who say they've never had a problem with chocolate but now, at 39, they can clear a box of truffles in one sitting. Of course, I suggest the S Factor diet.

You Don't Need Drugs

Doctors already know the power of serotonin. Anti-depressant drugs such as Prozac and Citalopram are known as selective serotonin re-uptake inhibitors (SSRIs). They work to lift depression by prolonging and amplifying the effect serotonin has on the brain. But, SSRIs can have side effects. You can feel groggy and your sex drive can be affected.

The reason serotonin is important for losing weight is because low serotonin not only makes you feel depressed, angry, tearful and so on, it also makes you feel HUNGRY, hence the PMS munchies! But the right level of serotonin helps reduce stress and anxiety and is a natural appetite suppressant. It also promotes sleep and that's good news for leptin levels, which you can read about later in this chapter (see page 17).

For dieters, then, serotonin is the all-round, all-natural diet miracle "pill". It turns down the volume of cravings, melts away emotional eating and basically makes you want to eat less. And the best bit is you can make it yourself for free!

Serotonin is made from the amino acid tryptophan, which you get from the food you eat. The best food sources of tryptophan include:

• Avocados
• Bananas
• Beans
• Chicken
• Eggs
• Fish
• Turkey

However, tryptophan is a small molecule and doesn't easily enter the brain. Once you have eaten sufficient tryptophan-containing foods, you also need a bit of sugar to stimulate the release of the hormone insulin. This helps tryptophan get into the brain and do its job. This doesn't mean you stuff yourself with Dairy Milk, but sweet things are not banned on the S Factor diet. Hooray!

. . . .

To find out if you may be low in serotonin, turn to the questionnaire on page 20.

Leptin

The "I'm-Not-Hungry" Hormone

Some of the most interesting research into why certain people gain weight and others don't has focused on hormones produced by our own fat. These include metabolic hormones such as leptin and adiponectin. Leptin is the one we know most about. It tells our brains when we have enough body fat, triggers a drop in appetite and speeds up metabolism – burning up excess body fat in the process. Interestingly, leptin is also important for fertility, which is one reason why seemingly cruel doctors often tell IVF candidates they need to lose weight. They are not just being sizeist!

Leptin production follows a circadian rhythm, that is, it rises and falls over a 24-hour cycle. Peak production of leptin is at night, so if you work night shifts, travel through different time zones or have a young baby who keeps you awake in the wee hours, you may develop leptin problems and gain weight.

There are two problems with leptin that could be causing you to gain weight: leptin depletion, in which your fat cells can't produce leptin, and more commonly, leptin resistance, in which you produce a high level of leptin but it doesn't have the normal effect of telling you that you're full. In both cases, your brain thinks you're starving, so it increases your appetite and slows down your metabolism – when actually your jeans are getting tighter and tighter.

Conquer Your Appetite

The clearest indication that you may have an issue with leptin is feeling constantly hungry. Gaining fat round your middle is also a symptom. However, the symptoms of leptin depletion and resistance can also mirror those for polycystic ovarian syndrome (PCOS). These symptoms include spots and/or excess hair along your jaw line,

disrupted periods and poor blood sugar control – which you can spot if you feel dizzy or irritable when you don't eat regularly. Also, look out for skin tags (benign growths) and something called Acanthosis Nigricans (AN). I had a client who showed me a sort of dark staining on her skin under her armpits. This was classic AN. It can also appear around your neck or in skin folds.

It's a nightmare chicken and egg situation, where you need to lose weight to tackle leptin problems, but leptin problems make it difficult to lose weight. The answer? The S Factor diet, of course!

No specific foods help us make leptin. However, foods rich in resistant starch, such as oats, can help those with leptin issues, as resistant starch speeds up your metabolism and reduces your appetite. You can also utilize other appetite-controlling hormones, such as ghrelin. Ghrelin levels increase before meals and go down again after meals. One way to reduce ghrelin is to stretch the stomach by eating high-volume foods (those with high water and high fibre content). The best foods to stabilize leptin include:

- Beans
- Eggs and lean protein
- Green bananas
- Nuts and seeds
- Oats
- Oily fish

. . . .

To find out if you have a leptin issue, turn to the questionnaire on page 21.

Dopamine

The "High-Motivation" Hormone

Dopamine has a variety of functions in the body, playing a role in processes ranging from behaviour and cognition to heart rate and blood pressure. In terms of your weight, dopamine is essential as it can boost motivation, focus and impulse control. It's also important for controlling "anticipatory pleasure" – or in other words, wanting something. Low levels of dopamine are associated with cravings. Good levels of dopamine help you stick to your diet, get you up and off to the gym and help you to plan and track your eating.

Dopamine production can be stimulated by drugs such as caffeine, nicotine, alcohol, cocaine and amphetamines, or even by falling in love. Sugary, fatty foods also hit the dopamine pathway in our brains. Less well-known is that adrenaline-fuelled activities such as extreme sports (bungee jumping "springs" to mind) can also push up dopamine levels. Those weird people who break records by repeatedly riding roller coasters may be subconsciously trying to balance their dopamine.

Beat the Sugar Rush

Riding the big dipper doesn't sound too bad. However, chronic spiking of dopamine levels can result in you needing more and more of it to feel good. This can disrupt your eating habits as you end up eating more and more sugary, fatty foods to satisfy your cravings.

Low levels of dopamine may be responsible for compulsive behaviour and/or addictions (see page 15). Many of my clients had a history of club drugs in their teens, or an extreme work life in their twenties and now can't stick to a diet. An American study published in 2010 in the respected *Journal of Obesity* confirmed a direct link between low dopamine levels and overeating.

Low dopamine is also associated with Attention Deficit Hyperactivity Disorder (ADHD). We know this is under-reported in adults and I often see clients who I think display traits of the disorder, including a lack of attention span and restlessness. They may also have a history of failed diets.

The key to good dopamine levels is prevention rather than cure. That is, you want to avoid over-stimulation of the dopamine pathway in the brain. If you already have an issue with dopamine, the best course of action is a combination of reducing stimulants such as tea, coffee and sugar, and eating foods that contain the raw material needed to produce dopamine.

Dopamine is made from tyrosine. The best food sources of tyrosine include:

- Almonds
- Bananas
- Fish
- Soy
- Watermelon

To find out if you have a dopamine issue, turn to the questionnaire on page 22.

Adrenals

The "Stress" Hormones

The adrenals are a pair of glands that sit on top of your kidneys. They pump out hormones such as adrenaline and cortisol in response to stress. This is important for your weight because too many of these hormones, in particular cortisol, cause you to store fat – especially in the dreaded muffin-top area.

Adrenal hormones can be stimulated by two types of stress: reactive and chronic. Reactive stress is caused by a particular event. For example, when you attempt to cross the road and a car comes screeching around the corner. Your heart pounds, your palms become sweaty and you may even feel slightly shaky. You may also shout something unmentionable at the driver because you experience a surge of aggression. Chronic stress is the low-level kind and sources can include bullying at work, a bad relationship, a long history of low self-esteem, being a worrier or being anxious about life in general. When you experience low-level anxiety, you feel fidgety and irritable, perhaps tired and slightly tearful. Your sleep may be disrupted. Most of all, you feel HUNGRY.

Keep Calm and Carry On

The stress/hunger connection is caused by over-activity in the deep limbic area of the brain – the area where emotional stress is processed. You may crave foods like chocolate that increase serotonin to compensate.

The adrenals are also responsible for salt balance in the body. When you are under stress, you may not only overeat, you may also crave salty, high-calorie foods such as peanuts or crisps. Plus, and here's the flubby tummy double whammy – stress also makes you store more of the food you eat as body fat. Sorry....

It starts well enough. You have two types of fat: white and brown. White fat manufactures certain hormones such as leptin. Brown fat contains B3 receptors which are stimulated by adrenaline. Brown fat in turn stimulates something called thermogenesis (the burning of calories to produce body heat). So, a bit of stress may help you lose weight.

However, chronic stress has been associated with a severely high level of cortisol and increased fat storage. This unbalances blood sugar and leads to higher levels of adrenaline. More adrenaline means more cortisol and more fat storage and round and round it goes as you quietly inflate. But the story doesn't end there. Once you gain weight, fat cells called adipokines act on the adrenals to produce yet more cortisol. This causes you to gain more weight, leading to more adipokines. Arrrgh!

The good news is that eating the right foods can help. First you need to keep your blood sugar stable to prevent overproduction of adrenaline and cortisol. Eating protein at every meal and minimizing carbs, especially sugar, is an excellent start. Your adrenals also require a wide variety of minerals, found in nuts, seeds and essential fats. Antioxidants and magnesium from colourful and dark-green veggies, and vitamin C in dark berries are also great. The best foods to nourish the adrenals include:

- Dark berries
- Dark-green and brightly coloured vegetables
- Nuts and seeds
- Oily fish
- Sea vegetables like nori seaweed

To find out if stress is causing you to gain weight, turn to the questionnaire on page 23.

Questionnaires

You may already have an inkling about which S Factor hormones you need to balance in order to lose weight, but the following questionnaires will really nail it down for you. So just answer the questions, add up your scores and you'll be ready to choose which meal plan will be most successful for you.

Serotonin

Consider each of the following statements and rate yourself on a scale of 1–5, with **1: strongly disagree, 2: disagree, 3: not sure, 4: agree and 5: strongly agree.**

1 I sometimes feel down or depressed.
2 I crave bread, pasta, cake, chocolate or wine, especially at night.
3 I don't sleep well.
4 After a hard day, I want to "treat" myself with food.
5 I am an emotional or comfort eater.
6 I really struggle on high-protein diets.
7 I am not hungry at breakfast time.
8 In the week before my period, I turn into a chocolate monster.
9 I am aged 38–55 (rate yourself 5 if true and 1 if false).
10 I tend to put on a spare tyre in the winter.

Results
Add up your scores. If you scored 30 or more out of 50, you may find it easier to lose weight if you balance your serotonin levels. Choose the Serotonin Plan (see pages 32–33) and look for recipes marked with an S.

Leptin

Consider each of the following statements and rate yourself on a scale of 1–5, with **1: strongly disagree, 2: disagree, 3: not sure, 4: agree** and **5: strongly agree.**

1 I feel hungry all the time.
2 I have a blood pressure of 130/80 or above (rate yourself 5 if true and 1 if false).
3 I have been diagnosed with type 2 diabetes (rate yourself 5 if true and 1 if false).
4 I gain weight round my middle.
5 I am more than 13kg (2st) overweight (rate yourself 5 if true and 1 if false).
6 I have new stretch marks, skin tags or Acanthosis Nigricans (AN) – see page 17.
7 I work shifts, travel a great deal or have small children who disrupt my sleep.
8 I suffer from spots/excess hair along my jaw line.
9 I crave bulky foods like pasta, rice and potatoes.
10 I know I need to lose weight, but however little I eat, I don't lose weight.

Results

Add up your scores. If you scored 30 or more out of 50, you may find it easier to lose weight if you balance your leptin levels. Choose the Leptin Plan (see pages 34–35) and look for recipes marked with an L.

"These questionnaires are designed to establish if you are generally low in all your S Factor hormones, or you have a particular issue with one or two of them."

Dopamine

Consider each of the following statements and rate yourself on a scale of 1–5, with **1: strongly disagree, 2: disagree, 3: not sure, 4: agree and 5: strongly agree.**

1 I start diets well but always fall off them.
2 Even if I am on a diet, if I see something "naughty" I can't say no.
3 I am an "all or nothing" person.
4 I like roller coasters, running marathons or computer games with lots of adrenaline-filled action.
5 I drink a lot of tea, coffee or diet cola.
6 I crave cake, chocolate or ice cream.
7 I think I work well under pressure and I am really good in a crisis.
8 I am a doer, rather than a thinker.
9 I sometimes prefer to be on my own.
10 I have a family history of alcohol/drugs/gambling/infidelity/ADHD (rate yourself 5 if true and 1 if false).

Results

Add up your scores. If you scored 30 or more out of 50, you may find it easier to lose weight if you balance your dopamine levels. Choose the Dopamine Plan (see pages 36–37) and look for recipes marked with a D.

. . . .

You are not a number

Most of us don't fit into neat little boxes, thank goodness. If you scored highly in more than one questionnaire (or in all of them), that's completely normal. Often in the world of hormones, it never rains but it pours.

If you have scored highly in more than one questionnaire, read the advice at the bottom of page 23 to find the perfect plan for you.

Adrenals

Consider each of the following statements and rate yourself on a scale of 1–5, with **1: strongly disagree, 2: disagree, 3: not sure, 4: agree** and **5: strongly agree.**

1 I have experienced redundancy, a break-up, money problems or bereavement over the last two years.
2 I fall asleep on buses/trains/at the hairdressers.
3 I sometimes lack patience, snap at those I love and then feel guilty about it.
4 I need caffeine, nicotine or sugar to get me going in the morning.
5 I feel tired at about 6pm, but get a second wind at about 10pm and often stay up late for some "me" time.
6 I am a worrier.
7 I get headaches/stomach aches for no apparent reason.
8 I have recurrent ear, nose and throat infections, thrush or mouth ulcers.
9 I have had one or more panic attacks, or am aware of a fast heart beat.
10 I feel calm after eating a big meal.

Results

Add up your scores. If you scored 30 or more out of 50, you may find it easier to lose weight if you balance your adrenal levels. Choose the Adrenals Plan (see pages 38–39) and look for recipes marked with an A.

. . . .

Choose the Serotonin Plan (see pages 32–33) if:
• you scored highly on the Serotonin and Dopamine questionnaires
• you scored highly on the Serotonin and Adrenals questionnaires

. . . .

Choose the Adrenals Plan (see pages 38–39) if:
• you scored highly on the Leptin and Adrenals questionnaires
• you scored highly on the Dopamine and Adrenals questionnaires

Choose the Leptin Plan (see pages 34–35) if:
• you scored highly on the Serotonin and Leptin questionnaires
• you scored highly on the Dopamine and Leptin questionnaires
• you scored highly on all of the S Factor hormone questionnaires

The Truth about Cravings

The biggest cause of failure on most diets is cravings. While the S Factor diet will help you to control hormone-induced cravings, it's important to remember there may also be specific foods and habits that make it harder for you to resist that morning choccy bar, freshly baked loaf of bread or tempting cheesecake, and you should consider these pitfalls before you start the diet.

Gluten "Fix"

When you eat gluten, a protein found in wheat, rye, barley and to a lesser extent in oats, spelt and kamut, it is broken down in your gut. This produces opioid peptides called gluteomorphins. The "morphins" bit is a clue. Heroin is a morphine. Of course the morphines you get from a slice (or four) of bread are much weaker. Still, they cross the blood-brain barrier and affect your brain. This is why so many of us have a muffin, or a bite of cake, or one spoonful of porridge and can't seem to stop. It's why we binge and fall off a diet when we succumb to a teeny bit of pasta. It gives us a "high".

Dairy Disasters

Dairy products can have a similar diet-destroying effect. The dairy protein casein, found in highest concentration in cow's milk products, breaks down to casomorphins. Cheese, another food that many of my clients absolutely love, has the highest concentration and thus gives the biggest high.

So, why can some people (supermodels and the like) nibble elegantly on the outer reaches of the cheese board, while others (the rest of us) want to clear it completely?

Histamine "High"

Histamine is a hormone we release when we encounter something our bodies don't tolerate well. It acts as a stimulant, so it too gives us a bit of a lift. Some people, referred to as "high-histamine individuals", naturally produce more histamine than others. High histamine seems to run in families and these families are described as "atopic". Asthma, eczema or hay fever are all atopic indicators. If you love wheat and dairy foods, that's another clue – you're craving the histamine high. If you often wake in the morning with a stuffy, snuffly or sneezy nose (allergic rhinitis), that's also a sign that you may be atopic.

So, if a high-histamine person eats a cheese sandwich (a gluteomorphins and casomorphins bomb!) they get a triple high – two times morphines and one times histamine. No wonder they want another sandwich. A low-histamine person simply doesn't get the same "kerpowee!" effect, and will be able to walk away from the fridge.

If you think you may be a high-histamine individual, you may be fighting a losing battle with gluten and casein and it may be best to avoid them completely. I always advise clients to go grain-free and dramatically reduce their dairy intake for the first two weeks of any diet. This gives them the opportunity to "free" themselves of any compulsive behaviour connected to these foods. It is perfectly possible to be gluten-free and dairy-free. Lots of gluten-free and dairy-free products are now available in supermarkets. Many of the S Factor recipes also feature alternative flours such as soy or chickpea flour, and non-dairy proteins like soy milk and tofu to help you along the way.

Chocolate Cravings

There is something special about chocolate and not just the taste. It not only hooks us with its silky combination of sugar and fat, it also contains other addictive chemicals. Number one is caffeine. A small Kit Kat has 5mg of caffeine, not huge compared to the 100mg in a cup of strong coffee, but it doesn't stop there. Chocolate contains a big whack of another stimulant, theobromine. It also contains phenylethylamine (PEA), another amphetamine-like substance and a little smidge of tetrahydrocannabinol (THC) – the active ingredient in marijuana!

Addicted to Dopamine

As I've explained, some people are genetically programmed to have fewer DRD2 dopamine receptors in their brain and seek to overstimulate the ones they do have with lots of sugary, fatty foods (see pages 15 and 18). If you have struggled to give up smoking or you go out for one drink and the rest of the night becomes a blur, it could be a clue that you have a DRD2 issue. You're a compulsive "all or nothing" kind of person with no "off switch".

In terms of diet, those with fewer DRD2 dopamine receptors will particularly crave high-fat, high-sugar combinations (cake, biscuits, chocolate and so on) because they most effectively stimulate the dopamine pathway. In the short term, eating four cream-filled doughnuts will help you stimulate your dopamine pathway and feel good. In the long term, you'll hate the way you look in a bikini.

The most important thing I have learnt from working with clients who use food compulsively is that you can't just take their favourite "drug" away. If you do, they will just flip to another compulsive behaviour. On a physical level they may crave the "high" that a chocolate bar gives them. On a psychological level, they may really miss the "zone out" that a big bowl of pasta delivers. You need to replace, not simply remove.

The good news is that there are other ways to stimulate DRD2 dopamine receptors. Exercise (the "runner's high"), love, sex and friendship all do it. I used to chain-smoke and eat piles of chocolate. Now I eat tofu and go to the gym everyday. Am I a saint? No. I simply know that if I don't get my DRD2 dopamine receptors bouncing like Tigger on a Stairmaster, I will be prey to any passing chocolate pusher.

Childhood Memories

There can also be an emotional trigger driving your cravings. For instance, if as a child you were given a sweet to soothe a sore knee, this sets up a link in your mind between pain (emotional as well as physical) and the "solution" – sugar. If you were taken out for cake as a "treat", this has taught you that food is a reward. So now you're an adult, you come home after a heavy work day and reward yourself with a family-sized tiramisu.

You can help yourself by identifying the foods you were conditioned to eat as a child and how you use food now. Is food a treat, a comfort or does it ease your anxiety? Once you know your programmed pitfalls, rather than turning to food when you're unhappy or stressed, play "Name That Emotion" instead. Ask yourself what emotion you are feeling and then say it out loud: "I AM ANGRY!", "I AM SAD". It's very freeing – and kind to your waistline.

The Truth about Night Eating

If you need to balance your S Factor hormones, evenings can be a battle with cravings. Dinner just wasn't enough, so you go foraging for chocolate, biscuits, cheese etc. There are a few reasons for this seemingly crazy behaviour:

You Need a Good Night's Sleep

If you're craving sweet things, this may be your body's way of trying to help you get a good night's sleep. Serotonin not only makes us feel calmer and happier, it also helps us sleep. Now, serotonin is made of protein, but as we know, you need a hit of the hormone insulin (which is stimulated by eating sugar) to actually get it to the brain.

Eating serotonin-balancing, sugary foods at night is like taking a natural sleeping pill. Trying to resist the urge to treat yourself with that biscuit after dinner is a losing battle. Plus, if you do succeed, it might be a case of win the battle, but lose the war. Poor sleep has been shown to stimulate appetite and cause weight gain. When you're exhausted you eat to give yourself energy, so you end up fat and knackered. Brilliant! In my experience, it's far better for those who are low in serotonin to satisfy their sweet craving in a controlled way with a small, sweet hit about an hour before bedtime. This is the only time when you go high GI (the higher the better), so ingredients like raisins and bananas are best.

Your Body is Starving

It's not often that we crave a can of tuna at night, to be fair, but many modern "healthy" diets can starve our bodies of the protein they need to function properly. This is why a protein-based snack at night can be useful as a way to manufacture more dopamine. Body builders eat cottage cheese before bed to prevent muscular tissue being broken down overnight. That's a bit extreme, but having a protein-rich drink before bed will help to stabilize your blood sugar.

Your Appetite "Off Switch" isn't Working

If you have become leptin resistant or are low in leptin, you may be craving food at night as a way of trying to stretch your stomach to activate other appetite-controlling hormones. You are looking for the appetite "off switch". And no, telling yourself you've just had dinner doesn't work. Far better to build in a low-calorie/high-volume snack such as a few vegetable sticks and a little houmous to ease those leptin munchies.

You're Stressed Out

Night-time eating can be an attempt to relieve anxiety. If you think about it, chewing is like squeezing a stress ball. It is a repetitive clenching and relaxing of your muscles which can also be a mental distraction from worries. The foods you choose may have a tranquilizing effect. To feel calmer, boost your intake of adrenal-friendly foods such as nuts and seeds before bed.

Most diets treat night eating like it's a cardinal sin. My experience with clients suggests that diets are more successful if you can have a snack at night. There is no magic about night eating – the calories aren't cursed. What is important is your calorie intake over a 24-hour period. If you want to save some of those calories for a night-time snack, no problem. The S Factor diet lets you do just that.

The S Factor Storecupboard

I wanted the S Factor diet to be as "unweird" as possible. I've taken everyday recipes and replaced some common ingredients that cause weight gain with ones that will balance your S Factor hormones and help you lose weight.

Flours

Almond Flour/Ground Almonds – a non-grain flour that works for cakes, biscuits and pastry bases. It's rich in essential fats but high in calories, so don't go mad with it.

Chickpea Flour – higher in protein than wheat flour, this is good for all your S Factor hormones as it contains resistant starch. Resistant starch speeds up your metabolism and reduces your appetite. It also helps stabilize blood sugar.

Polenta – a bit high GI, but it makes the best non-wheat crumb for chicken or fish, and also makes delicious muffins.

Rye Flour – much lower in gluten than wheat.

Soya flour – this flour is very high in protein which means it's great for keeping blood sugar balanced and preventing fat storage. If you are concerned about possible GM contamination, you could use quinoa flour instead.

Sweeteners

You won't be trowelling sugar onto your S Factor meals, and I don't use honey in any of my recipes either. Although honey is a natural sweetener (and in the case of Manuka honey, it's even antibacterial), it spikes blood sugar which is a disaster for your S Factor hormones. Instead, I use:

Agave Syrup – a good stand-in syrup for pancakes and desserts. Agave syrup (also known as agave nectar) is made from a type of cactus. It tastes lovely and sweet, but it doesn't lift blood sugar.

Stevia – white and granular like sugar, stevia is made from the leaf of a small Paraguayan shrub. In its concentrated form it's 300–400 times sweeter than sugar. It's usually sold mixed with sucralose so you can still use it spoon for spoon like sugar. It doesn't raise blood sugar and it's also calorie free.

Xylitol – also white and granular like sugar, xylitol is a sugar alcohol that is extracted from plants and trees. It has 40% fewer calories than sugar and doesn't raise blood sugar. Check the packet carefully though, as xylitol made from corn can taste minty. Xylitol made from birch trees is a much better option for sauces and baking.

Other S Factor Stars

Fermented Soy – A fantastic low-fat vegetarian protein food, but you need to be careful. Too much soy (especially the modern manufactured kind found in mass-produced soya milk and yogurts) can disrupt thyroid function. An underactive thyroid is a recipe for weight gain. Vegetarians should stick to fermented soy products like miso and tempeh.

Unripe Bananas – high in resistant starch, eating bananas is a brilliant way to help leptin levels. Pick unripe or even green ones, as ripe bananas can unbalance blood sugar.

Secrets of Success

Starting the S Factor diet is either going to feel fantastically exciting (hopefully) or a bit daunting. You're putting yourself on the road to a slimmer, healthier, happier future, but you may also feel a teeny bit apprehensive.

Perhaps you're afraid of failure? If you're a yo-yo dieter, you might have a history of failed diets and worry you won't succeed. Perhaps you're scared of change? The S Factor diet is a gear shift for most people. If you're used to having toast and jam for breakfast, a bowl of sugary cereal or nothing at all, then life will not be quite the same.

Maybe you're grieving? Starting the S Factor diet means you have to say goodbye to some old food habits – that coffee break muffin or in-car chocolate treat, perhaps? You and I know that these weren't helpful, but they may have served a purpose in relieving boredom or easing stress or loneliness and it can feel sad to give them up. They have been a friend as well as a foe.

The thing to remember is that as you progress, your S Factor hormones will rebalance and your cravings will ease. New habits will "bed in" and it will get easier and easier – plus you'll be feeling better and better!

Here's how to improve the odds that you'll make it to your goal weight and stay there.

Eat Three Square Meals (and One S Factor Snack) Per Day

Eating regularly helps you lose weight because it keeps your blood sugar and mood steady, and prevents sugar cravings turning you into the cookie monster! This doesn't mean you can attach yourself to the fridge with a piece of elastic. Constant snacking stops weight loss in its tracks.

Instead, you should aim to enjoy three healthy meals (and one S Factor snack) per day.

Breakfast – when you wake up, your blood sugar is low as you didn't eat while you were asleep (hopefully, although I have had clients who have done that!). Low blood sugar has two major effects on the body. Firstly, it makes your thinking foggy – so you are more likely to succumb to sugar cravings. Secondly, it can stimulate cortisol and cause fat storage – so you inhale a Danish pastry and it goes straight to your thighs. The key to fat loss is to stabilize blood sugar, which in turn will stabilize your appetite-reducing, fat-burning S Factor hormones. How do you do that? By eating a breakfast that's high in lean protein.

Lunch – some people panic at the idea of no daytime snacks, but go back a generation and there was no such thing as snack food and we were all a lot slimmer. The right lunch should carry you through to dinner time. Again, the way to make lunch last is to build it around healthy protein (like fish and lean meat) and vegetables. Add more vegetables if you're worried you'll be hungry later on.

Dinner – nobody wants diet food at dinner time. We want food that's as close to the meals we normally eat as possible. Problem is, that's probably the food which caused us to gain weight in the first place. And more often than not, it's comfort food: stodgy piles of potatoes, chips, pasta or rice. The challenge, then, is to substitute the mounds of what I call "white foods" (bread, rice, pasta, potatoes) for ones that are less fattening. So, the mash, rice and pasta in all the S Factor dinner recipes are made from vegetables, beans or pulses. You'll find many of these recipes are family meals because, in my experience, dieters are more successful when they can prepare the same meal for everyone. There's nothing worse then serving one delicious dish for your partner and children, and then eating diet gruel in the corner like Billy no-mates.

Dessert – the desire for something sweet is probably the number one reason why dieters fall off the wagon. On certain high-protein plans (mentioning no names!) even fruit is banned, and that's the sure-fire way to madness, cravings and bingeing. The S Factor solution is to give you a sweet treat after one of your meals (if you want one), but to substitute high-sugar, high-fat puds for ones that are higher in protein and lower in fat.

The S Factor Snack – eating the right snack at night can help all of your S Factor hormones. It's what makes this plan so effective.

Keep That Muffin Top Away
Here are some tips to help keep those skinny jeans zipped once you've reached your goal weight:
- **No second helpings** – put your meal on a plate and put any leftovers in storage containers immediately before you sit down to eat.
- **Don't graze** – only add in an afternoon snack if there is a gap of more than five hours between lunch and dinner or you're working out.

- **Exercise** – if you superglue yourself to the sofa once you get to your goal weight, your bottom will inflate.
- **Address your stress levels** – stress makes you fat, so make sure you take time to relax. Try yoga, tai chi or learn self-hypnosis and remember to get enough sleep.
- **Plan ahead** – pack your lunch; make sure you have the right food in the fridge; and choose the restaurant on a night out so you can research the menu first.
- **Don't buy things you shouldn't eat** – if you don't have biscuits, cakes and ice creams in your home, you won't eat them. If you have kids, make a rule that they only eat cakes and biscuits outside the house. Take them out to a café for the occasional sugar-fest, or buy them a treat on the way home from school.

Stop the rot
Of course, the wheels may come off every so often. You go on holiday and hit the all-inclusive buffet too hard, it's Christmas or your birthday… but have a 1.5kg (3lb) limit. If your weight goes up beyond that, pull in the reins. It's easier to shift 1.5kg (3lb) than 20kg (3st) – which is how much I always used to put back on!

Work Out What Works For You
Whatever helped you to lose the weight on the 14-day plan will also help you to keep it off. So analyze and write down which were the most important changes you made during Phases 1 and 2. If you batch cooked on a Sunday night while you were losing weight, for example, keep on doing it. These are your winning strategies for eating for life.

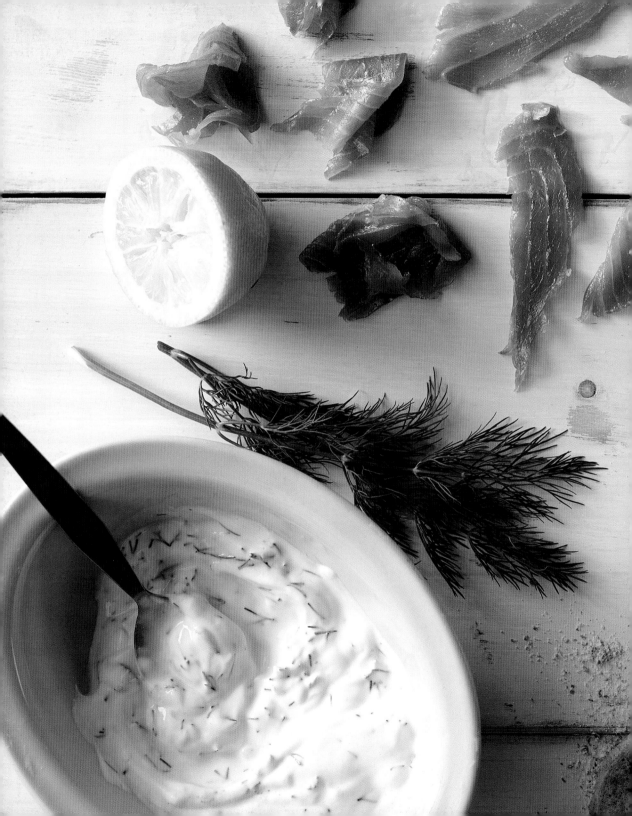

The S Factor 14-Day Diet

Rather than offering one standard meal plan, the
S Factor diet is tailored to work for you. Your questionnaire
results (see pages 20–23) should have revealed the right
S Factor hormone plan for you. Whichever plan you follow,
you could drop up to a dress size in two weeks.

Each plan is split into two stages. Phase 1 is the fast fat
attack stage, while Phase 2 focuses on steadier weight
loss and establishing your improved eating routine. If you
have more than a dress size to lose, you can stick with
Phase 2 until you reach your goal weight. If you're happy
to lose weight slowly, go straight to Phase 2. Ready?
Steady? Let's go!

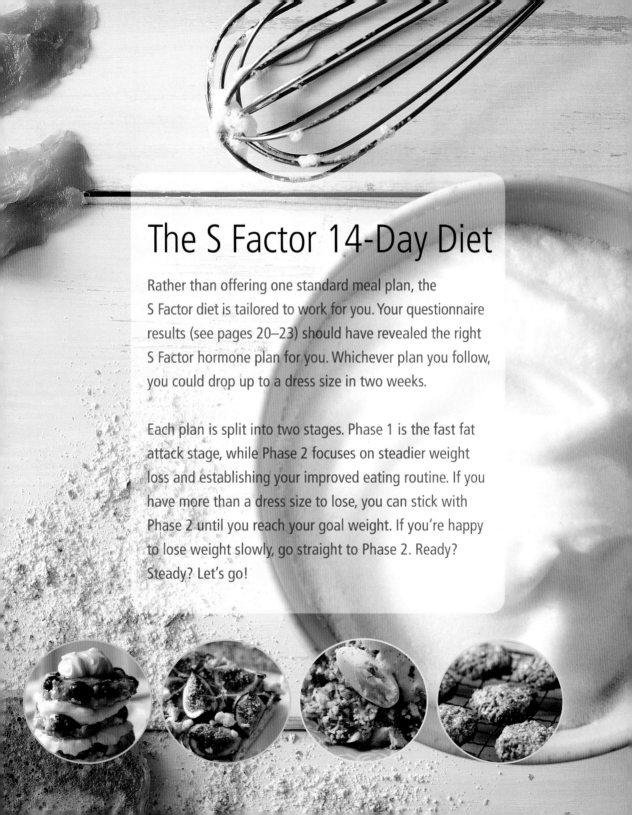

Serotonin Phase 1
7-Day Meal Plan

Phase 1 features few grains (bread, pasta, rice etc) or beans. This may seem daunting, but it will cut calories, encourage you to experiment with new foods, and, most importantly, balance serotonin.

DAY 1
Breakfast California Superfood Omelette (see page 47)
Lunch Thai Hot & Sour Seafood Soup (see page 59)
Dinner Moroccan Tagine with Broccoli & Pistachio "Tabbouleh" (see page 78), Raspberry Granita (see page 95)
S Factor Snack Spiced Hot Chocolate (see page 120)

DAY 2
Breakfast Grilled Portobello Mushrooms with Roasted Vine Tomatoes (see page 48)
Lunch Vietnamese Mussels (see page 65)
Dinner Spinach & Cheese "Cannelloni" (see page 91), Greek Quinces (see page 98)
S Factor Snack Spiced Hot Chocolate (see page 120)

DAY 3
Breakfast Smoked Haddock Vedgerie (see page 53)
Lunch Cantonese Pork in Chicory Spoons (see page 57)
Dinner Fig & Feta Tart (see page 92), Champagne Jellies (see page 96)
S Factor Snack Spiced Hot Chocolate (see page 120)

DAY 4
Breakfast California Superfood Omelette (see page 47)
Lunch Vietnamese Mussels (see page 65)
Dinner Cretan Turkey Stew (see page 76), Japanese Fruit Salad (see page 96)
S Factor Snack Spiced Hot Chocolate (see page 120)

DAY 5
Breakfast Grilled Portobello Mushrooms with Roasted Vine Tomatoes (see page 48)
Lunch Sicilian Artichoke & Egg "Pizzas" (see page 68)
Dinner Keralan Prawn Curry with Lime & Coriander "Rice" (see page 88), Raspberry Granita (see page 95)
S Factor Snack Spiced Hot Chocolate (see page 120)

DAY 6
Breakfast Smoked Haddock Vedgerie (see page 53)
Lunch Thai Hot & Sour Seafood Soup (see page 59)
Dinner Pollock with Salsa Verde & Carrot Purée (see page 87), Coconut Sorbet (see page 95)
S Factor Snack Spiced Hot Chocolate (see page 120)

DAY 7
Breakfast California Superfood Omelette (see page 47)
Lunch Courgette "Tagliatelle" (see page 70)
Dinner Spinach & Cheese "Cannelloni" (see page 91), Cherry & Almond Clafoutis (see page 102)
S Factor Snack Spiced Hot Chocolate (see page 120)

Serotonin Phase 2
7-Day Meal Plan

Phase 2 still contains plenty of protein so that you can make serotonin. It also includes more carbs to help the serotonin reach your brain so you can lose weight and feel great.

DAY 1
Breakfast Blueberry Pancake Stacks (see page 42)
Lunch Thai Hot & Sour Seafood Soup (see page 59)
Dinner Steak Puttanesca with Parmesan Brussels Sprouts (see page 83), Raspberry Granita (see page 95)
S Factor Snack Banana Rice Pudding (see page 108)

DAY 2
Breakfast Grilled Portobello Mushrooms with Roasted Vine Tomatoes (see page 48)
Lunch Tartelettes Niçoises (see page 60)
Dinner Polenta-Crusted Chicken with Cauliflower "Mash" (see page 75), Cherry & Almond Clafoutis (see page 102)
S Factor Snack Blackberry Yogurt Lollies (see page 107)

DAY 3
Breakfast Fruity Yogurt Crunch (see page 44)
Lunch Cantonese Pork in Chicory Spoons (see page 57)
Dinner Pollock with Salsa Verde & Carrot Purée (see page 87), Coconut Sorbet (see page 95)
S Factor Snack Indian-Style Trail Mix (see page 118)

DAY 4
Breakfast California Superfood Omelette (see p 47)
Lunch Mini Feta-Stuffed Lamb Burgers with Polenta Muffins (see page 58)
Dinner Keralan Prawn Curry with Lime & Coriander "Rice" (see page 88), Japanese Fruit Salad (see page 96)
S Factor Snack Rainbow Macaroons (see page 114)

DAY 5
Breakfast Cowboy Breakfast (see page 49)
Lunch Courgette "Tagliatelle" (see page 70)
Dinner Shepherd's Pie (see page 79), Champagne Jellies (see page 96)
S Factor Snack Chilli Pitta Crisps (see page 118)

DAY 6
Breakfast Smoked Haddock Vedgerie (see page 53)
Lunch Chicken with Puy Lentils (see page 54)
Dinner Braised Lamb Shanks with Lentil & Rosemary Mash (see page 81), Raspberry Granita (see page 95)
S Factor Snack Banana, Apple & Walnut Bread (see page 117)

DAY 7
Breakfast Buckwheat Blinis with Smoked Salmon & Lemon Crème Fraîche (see page 50)
Lunch Vietnamese Mussels (see page 65)
Dinner Cretan Turkey Stew (see page 76), Apple & Blueberry Crumble with Vanilla Tofu Ice Cream (see page 101)
S Factor Snack Chocolate Yogurt Mousses (see page 109)

Leptin Phase 1
7-Day Meal Plan

Phase 1 is based around lean protein and high-volume, low-cal foods – that is to say vegetables. To help you feel full, it also includes grains like oats, which are a good source of resistant starch.

DAY 1

Breakfast Fruity Yogurt Crunch (see page 44)

Lunch Mini Feta-Stuffed Lamb Burgers with Polenta Muffins (see page 58)

Dinner Polenta-Crusted Chicken with Cauliflower "Mash" (see page 75), Raspberry Granita (see page 95)

S Factor Snack Apricot & Oat Cookies (see page 112)

DAY 2

Breakfast Sunflower Seed Breakfast Loaf (see page 41)

Lunch Moroccan Chickpea Balls with Beetroot Dip (see page 69)

Dinner Pollock with Salsa Verde & Carrot Purée (see page 87), Japanese Fruit Salad (see page 96)

S Factor Snack Apricot & Oat Cookies (see page 112)

DAY 3

Breakfast Buckwheat Blinis with Smoked Salmon & Lemon Crème Fraîche (see page 50)

Lunch Chicken with Puy Lentils (see page 54)

Dinner Steak Puttanesca with Parmesan Brussels Sprouts (see page 83), Coconut Sorbet (see page 95)

S Factor Snack Apricot & Oat Cookies (see page 112)

DAY 4

Breakfast Cowboy Breakfast (see page 49)

Lunch Tiger Prawns with Cauliflower "Couscous" (see page 63)

Dinner Shepherd's Pie (see page 79), Champagne Jellies (see page 96)

S Factor Snack Apricot & Oat Cookies (see page 112)

DAY 5

Breakfast Sunflower Seed Breakfast Loaf (see page 41)

Lunch Middle Eastern Broad Bean & Brown Rice Soup (see page 66)

Dinner Keralan Prawn Curry with Lime & Coriander "Rice" (see page 88), Greek Quinces (see page 98)

S Factor Snack Apricot & Oat Cookies (see page 112)

DAY 6

Breakfast Fruity Yogurt Crunch (see page 44)

Lunch Tartelettes Niçoises (see page 60)

Dinner Salmon Fishcakes with Parsley Sauce & Fresh Minted Peas (see page 84), Raspberry Granita (see page 95)

S Factor Snack Apricot & Oat Cookies (see page 112)

DAY 7

Breakfast Buckwheat Blinis with Smoked Salmon & Lemon Crème Fraîche (see page 50)

Lunch Courgette "Tagliatelle" (see page 70)

Dinner Polenta-Crusted Chicken with Cauliflower "Mash" (see page 75), Baked Café Mocha Cheesecake (see page 99)

S Factor Snack Apricot & Oat Cookies (see page 112)

Leptin Phase 2
7-Day Meal Plan

Phase 2 is still about high-volume, low-cal foods that will help you hang on to that feeling of fullness. And, in case you've been missing them, it also includes an extra portion of grains.

DAY 1
Breakfast Buckwheat Blinis with Smoked Salmon & Lemon Crème Fraîche (see page 50)

Lunch Middle Eastern Broad Bean & Brown Rice Soup (see page 66)

Dinner Catalan Seafood & Fennel Stew with Courgette Purée (see page 89), Apple & Blueberry Crumble with Vanilla Tofu Ice Cream (see page 101)

S Factor Snack Banana, Apple & Walnut Bread (see page 117)

DAY 2
Breakfast Quinoa Porridge with Apple & Raisins (see page 44)

Lunch Tartelettes Niçoises (see page 60)

Dinner Moroccan Tagine with Broccoli & Pistachio "Tabbouleh" (see page 78), Fig Flowers with Orange Flower Water (see page 98)

S Factor Snack Chilli Pitta Crisps (see page 118)

DAY 3
Breakfast Fruity Yogurt Crunch (see page 44)

Lunch Moroccan Chickpea Balls with Beetroot Dip (see page 69)

Dinner Steak Puttanesca with Parmesan Brussels Sprouts (see page 83), Greek Quinces (see page 98)

S Factor Snack Banana Rice Pudding (see page 108)

DAY 4
Breakfast Blueberry Pancake Stacks (see page 42)

Lunch Quinoa & Pine Nut Dolmades with Tzatziki (see page 73)

Dinner Braised Lamb Shanks with Lentil & Rosemary Mash (see page 81), Rhubarb Soufflés (see page 105)

S Factor Snack Indian-Style Trail Mix (see page 118)

DAY 5
Breakfast Sunflower Seed Breakfast Loaf (see page 41)

Lunch Courgette "Tagliatelle" (see page 70)

Dinner Shepherd's Pie (see page 79), Baked Café Mocha Cheesecake (see page 99)

S Factor Snack Chilli Pitta Crisps (see page 118)

DAY 6
Breakfast Cowboy Breakfast (see page 49)

Lunch Moroccan Chickpea Balls with Beetroot Dip (see page 69)

Dinner Steak Puttanesca with Parmesan Brussels Sprouts (see page 83), Fig Flowers with Orange Flower Water (see page 98)

S Factor Snack Banana Rice Pudding (see page 108)

DAY 7
Breakfast Buckwheat Blinis with Smoked Salmon & Lemon Crème Fraîche (see page 50)

Lunch Courgette "Tagliatelle" (see page 70)

Dinner Fig & Feta Tart (see page 92), Apple & Blueberry Crumble with Vanilla Tofu Ice Cream (see page 101)

S Factor Snack Indian-Style Trail Mix (see page 118)

Dopamine Phase 1
7-Day Meal Plan

Phase 1 is filled with delicious protein-rich recipes to help you balance your dopamine levels. Your meals will be based around lean protein, good fats and lots of veggies.

DAY 1

Breakfast California Superfood Omelette (see page 47)

Lunch Thai Hot & Sour Seafood Soup (see page 59)

Dinner Steak Puttanesca with Parmesan Brussels Sprouts (see page 83), Champagne Jellies (see page 96)

S Factor Snack Tangy Toasted Seeds (see page 119)

DAY 2

Breakfast Grilled Portobello Mushrooms with Roasted Vine Tomatoes (see page 48)

Lunch Mini Feta-Stuffed Lamb Burgers with Polenta Muffins (see page 58)

Dinner Spinach & Cheese "Cannelloni" (see page 91), Cherry & Almond Clafoutis (see page 102)

S Factor Snack Tangy Toasted Seeds (see page 119)

DAY 3

Breakfast Smoked Haddock Vedgerie (see page 53)

Lunch Cantonese Pork in Chicory Spoons (see page 57)

Dinner Polenta-Crusted Chicken with Cauliflower "Mash" (see page 75), Rhubarb Soufflés (see page 105)

S Factor Snack Tangy Toasted Seeds (see page 119)

DAY 4

Breakfast California Superfood Omelette (see page 47)

Lunch Tiger Prawns with Cauliflower "Couscous" (see page 63)

Dinner Cretan Turkey Stew (see page 76), Baked Café Mocha Cheesecake (page 99)

S Factor Snack Tangy Toasted Seeds (see page 119)

DAY 5

Breakfast Grilled Portobello Mushrooms with Roasted Vine Tomatoes (see page 48)

Lunch Sicilian Artichoke & Egg "Pizzas" (see page 68)

Dinner Spinach & Cheese "Cannelloni" (see page 91), Raspberry Granita (see page 95)

S Factor Snack Tangy Toasted Seeds (see page 119)

DAY 6

Breakfast Smoked Haddock Vedgerie (see page 53)

Lunch Vietnamese Mussels (see page 65)

Dinner Catalan Seafood & Fennel Stew with Courgette Purée (see page 89), Coconut Sorbet (see page 95)

S Factor Snack Tangy Toasted Seeds (see page 119)

DAY 7

Breakfast California Superfood Omelette (see page 47)

Lunch Tartelettes Niçoises (see page 60)

Dinner Pollock with Salsa Verde & Carrot Purée (see page 87), Champagne Jellies (see page 96)

S Factor Snack Tangy Toasted Seeds (see page 119)

Dopamine Phase 2
7-Day Meal Plan

Phase 2 sticks with the protein-rich breakfasts to keep your dopamine production under control. You'll also be able to have more beans and grains, and a little more fat.

DAY 1
Breakfast Sunflower Seed Breakfast Loaf (see page 41)
Lunch Sicilian Artichoke & Egg "Pizzas" (see page 68)
Dinner Polenta-Crusted Chicken with Cauliflower "Mash" (see page 75), Fig Flowers with Orange Flower Water (see page 98)
S Factor Snack Chocolate Yogurt Mousses (see page 109)

DAY 2
Breakfast Blueberry Pancake Stacks (see page 42)
Lunch Chicken with Puy Lentils (see page 54)
Dinner Moroccan Tagine with Broccoli & Pistachio "Tabbouleh" (see page 78), Japanese Fruit Salad (see page 96)
S Factor Snack Spiced Hot Chocolate (see page 120)

DAY 3
Breakfast Sunflower Seed Breakfast Loaf (see page 41)
Lunch Tiger Prawns with Cauliflower "Couscous" (see page 63)
Dinner Pollock with Salsa Verde & Carrot Purée (see page 87), Greek Quinces (see page 98)
S Factor Snack Banana, Apple & Walnut Bread (see page 117)

DAY 4
Breakfast Grilled Portobello Mushrooms with Roasted Vine Tomatoes (see page 48)
Lunch Thai Hot & Sour Seafood Soup (see page 59)
Dinner Polenta-Crusted Chicken with Cauliflower "Mash" (see page 75), Raspberry Granita (see page 95)
S Factor Snack Spiced Pecans (see page 119)

DAY 5
Breakfast California Superfood Omelette (see page 47)
Lunch Vietnamese Mussels (see page 65)
Dinner Keralan Prawn Curry with Lime & Coriander "Rice" (see page 88), Rhubarb Soufflés (see page 105)
S Factor Snack Old-Fashioned Lemon Cheesecakes (see page 111)

DAY 6
Breakfast Grilled Portobello Mushrooms with Roasted Vine Tomatoes (see page 48)
Lunch Cantonese Pork in Chicory Spoons (see page 57)
Dinner Catalan Seafood & Fennel Stew with Courgette Purée (see page 89), Cherry & Almond Clafoutis (see page 102)
S Factor Snack Barley Bedtime Drink (see page 120)

DAY 7
Breakfast Smoked Haddock Vedgerie (see page 53)
Lunch Mini Feta-Stuffed Lamb Burgers with Polenta Muffins (see page 58)
Dinner Spinach & Cheese "Cannelloni" (see page 91), Baked Café Mocha Cheesecake (see page 99)
S Factor Snack Blackberry Yogurt Lollies (see page 107)

Adrenals Phase 1
7-Day Meal Plan

Phase 1 of the adrenals plan is designed to balance your stress hormones. It's low in grains but includes plenty of hormone-balancing protein and brain-boosting healthy fats.

DAY 1
Breakfast Fruity Yogurt Crunch (see page 44)
Lunch Sicilian Artichoke & Egg "Pizzas" (see page 68)
Dinner Keralan Prawn Curry with Lime & Coriander "Rice" (see page 88), Coconut Sorbet (see page 95)
S Factor Snack Barley Bedtime Drink (see page 120)

DAY 2
Breakfast California Superfood Omelette (see page 47)
Lunch Thai Hot & Sour Seafood Soup (see page 59)
Dinner Moroccan Tagine with Broccoli & Pistachio "Tabbouleh" (see page 78), Fig Flowers with Orange Flower Water (see page 98)
S Factor Snack Barley Bedtime Drink (see page 120)

DAY 3
Breakfast Smoked Haddock Vedgerie (see page 53)
Lunch Vietnamese Mussels (see page 65)
Dinner Keralan Prawn Curry with Lime & Coriander "Rice" (see page 88), Baked Café Mocha Cheesecake (page 99)
S Factor Snack Barley Bedtime Drink (see page 120)

DAY 4
Breakfast Fruity Yogurt Crunch (see page 44)
Lunch Cantonese Pork in Chicory Spoons (see page 57)
Dinner Salmon Fishcakes with Parsley Sauce & Fresh Minted Peas (see page 84), Japanese Fruit Salad (see page 96)
S Factor Snack Barley Bedtime Drink (see page 120)

DAY 5
Breakfast Buckwheat Blinis with Smoked Salmon & Lemon Crème Fraîche (see page 50)
Lunch Thai Hot & Sour Seafood Soup (see page 59)
Dinner Pollock with Salsa Verde & Carrot Purée (see page 87), Fig Flowers with Orange Flower Water (see page 98)
S Factor Snack Barley Bedtime Drink (see page 120)

DAY 6
Breakfast California Superfood Omelette (see page 47)
Lunch Chicken with Puy Lentils (see page 54)
Dinner Spinach & Cheese "Cannelloni" (see page 91), Champagne Jellies (see page 96)
S Factor Snack Barley Bedtime Drink (see page 120)

DAY 7
Breakfast Sunflower Seed Breakfast Loaf (see page 41)
Lunch Courgette "Tagliatelle" (see page 70)
Dinner Catalan Seafood & Fennel Stew with Courgette Purée (see page 89), Cherry & Almond Clafoutis (see page 102)
S Factor Snack Barley Bedtime Drink (see page 120))

Adrenals Phase 2
7-Day Meal Plan

Phase 2 focuses on high-protein, mineral-rich meals. Although carbs are kept to a minimum to stabilize your blood sugar, this phase does introduce one extra portion of grains per day.

DAY 1

Breakfast Sunflower Seed Breakfast Loaf (see page 41)

Lunch Tartelettes Niçoises (see page 60)

Dinner Salmon Fishcakes with Parsley Sauce & Fresh Minted Peas (see page 84), Japanese Fruit Salad (see page 96)

S Factor Snack Banana, Apple & Walnut Bread (see page 117)

DAY 2

Breakfast Fruity Yogurt Crunch (see page 44)

Lunch Quinoa & Pine Nut Dolmades with Tzatziki (see page 73)

Dinner Fig & Feta Tart (see page 92), Rhubarb Soufflés (see page 105)

S Factor Snack Old-Fashioned Lemon Cheesecakes (see page 111)

DAY 3

Breakfast Quinoa Porridge with Apple & Raisins (see page 44)

Lunch Chicken with Puy Lentils (see page 54)

Dinner Catalan Seafood & Fennel Stew with Courgette Purée (see page 89), Baked Café Mocha Cheesecake (see page 99)

S Factor Snack Rainbow Macaroons (see page 114)

DAY 4

Breakfast California Superfood Omelette (see page 47)

Lunch Vietnamese Mussels (see page 65)

Dinner Spinach & Cheese "Cannelloni" (see page 91), Apple & Blueberry Crumble with Vanilla Tofu Ice Cream (see page 101)

S Factor Snack Apricot & Oat Cookies (see page 112)

DAY 5

Breakfast Smoked Haddock Vedgerie (see page 53)

Lunch Sicilian Artichoke & Egg "Pizzas" (see page 68)

Dinner Polenta-Crusted Chicken with Cauliflower Mash (see page 75), Japanese Fruit Salad (see page 96)

S Factor Snack Banana, Apple & Walnut Bread (see page 117)

DAY 6

Breakfast Sunflower Seed Breakfast Loaf (see page 41)

Lunch Moroccan Chickpea Balls with Beetroot Dip (see page 69)

Dinner Keralan Prawn Curry with Lime & Coriander "Rice" (see page 88), Baked Café Mocha Cheesecake (page 99)

S Factor Snack Tangy Toasted Seeds (see page 119)

DAY 7

Breakfast Buckwheat Blinis with Smoked Salmon & Lemon Crème Fraîche (see page 50)

Lunch Middle Eastern Broad Bean & Brown Rice Soup (see page 66)

Dinner Braised Lamb Shanks with Lentil & Rosemary Mash (see page 81), Raspberry Granita (see page 95)

S Factor Snack Spiced Pecans (see page 119)

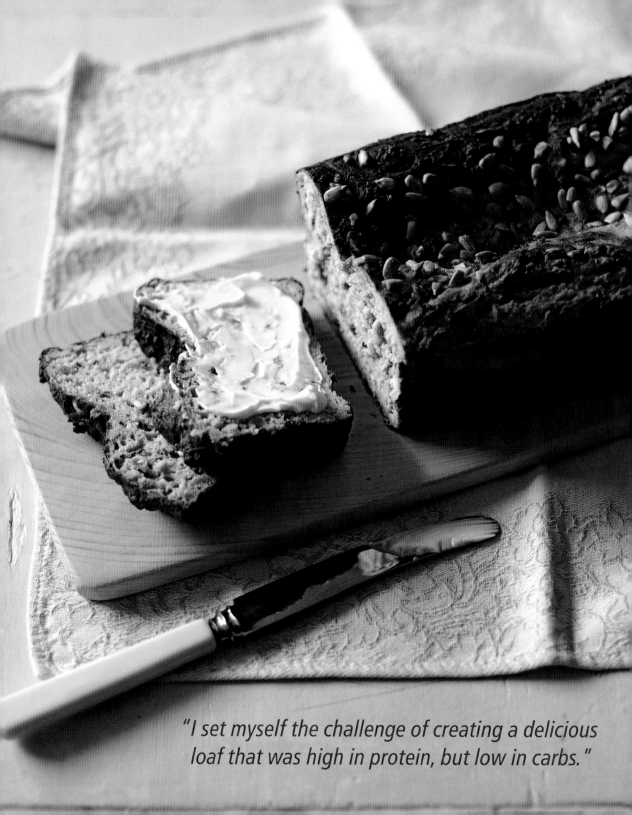

"I set myself the challenge of creating a delicious loaf that was high in protein, but low in carbs."

Sunflower Seed Breakfast Loaf

MAKES: 5 servings
PREPARATION TIME: 10 minutes
COOKING TIME: 40 minutes

I love bread, but it can be a slippery slope to a sugar binge. One slice is never enough. This cottage cheese, soya flour and egg white loaf (honestly, it tastes good) is now one of my favourite recipes. Slice and freeze it to help with portion control.

400g/14oz/scant 1⅔ cups reduced-fat cottage cheese
2 egg whites
120g/4¼oz/1 cup soya flour, sifted
2 tsp baking powder
2 tsp caraway seeds
a pinch of ground nutmeg
a pinch of ground cinnamon, plus extra for sprinkling (optional)
a pinch of fine sea salt
50g/1¾oz/scant ½ cup sunflower seeds, plus 1 tbsp extra for sprinkling
reduced-fat cream cheese, to serve

1 Preheat the oven to 160°C/315°F/Gas 2–3 and line a 450g/1lb loaf tin with baking parchment. Put the cottage cheese in a blender or food processor and process until a creamy paste forms. Transfer to a large bowl.

2 Whisk the egg whites in a clean bowl until they form soft peaks, then gently fold them into the cottage cheese, using a metal spoon.

3 Add all of the remaining ingredients and 1 tablespoon water and stir until well combined. Pour the dough into the tin and bake for 35–40 minutes until a skewer inserted in the centre comes out clean.

4 Turn the loaf out of the tin, transfer to a wire rack and leave to cool completely. Sprinkle with sunflower seeds and cut the loaf into 10 slices. Spread 1 teaspoon of cream cheese over each slice and serve sprinkled with cinnamon, if you like.

Nutritional analysis per serving: Calories 230kcal **Protein** 9.4g **Carbohydrates** 11.8g **Fat** 4.9g

Blueberry Pancake Stacks

MAKES: 4 servings
PREPARATION TIME: 5 minutes
COOKING TIME: 12 minutes

Many of us associate American-style pancakes with belly-busting hotel breakfast buffets, but they don't have to be fattening. I've tweaked the traditional recipe to make these pancakes, which are low in fat and high in protein to keep you feeling full. Plus, they're really quick and easy to make.

160g/5¾oz/scant 1⅔ cups rolled oats
250g/9oz/1 cup reduced-fat cottage cheese
4 eggs, beaten
1 tsp vanilla extract
250g/9oz blueberries, plus 90g/3¼oz extra to serve
extra virgin olive oil cooking spray
300g/10½oz/scant 1¼ cups reduced-fat Greek yogurt
4 tbsp agave syrup

1 Put the oats, cottage cheese, eggs and vanilla extract in a large mixing bowl and slowly beat together to make a thick, smooth batter. Using a large metal spoon, carefully fold in the blueberries, taking care not to break them up.

2 Preheat the oven to 100°C/200°F/Gas ½. Mist a non-stick frying pan with cooking spray and heat over a medium heat until it just starts to smoke. Working in batches, pour 1 tablespoon of the batter into the pan to make a pancake and repeat, spacing the pancakes slightly apart. Cook for 2–3 minutes on each side until the tops bubble and the edges of the pancakes start to brown. Transfer to a heatproof plate and keep warm in the oven while you repeat with the remaining batter to make 16 pancakes, misting the pan again with cooking spray if necessary.

3 To assemble a stack, top 1 pancake with 1 tablespoon of yogurt, then place another pancake on top followed by another 1 tablespoon of yogurt. Repeat the layers until you have a stack of 4 pancakes. Repeat with the remaining pancakes and yogurt to make 4 equal portions. Top the stacks with the remaining yogurt. Drizzle with agave syrup and serve with blueberries.

Nutritional analysis per serving: Calories 291.6kcal **Protein** 22.3g **Carbohydrates** 57.4g **Fat** 11.8g

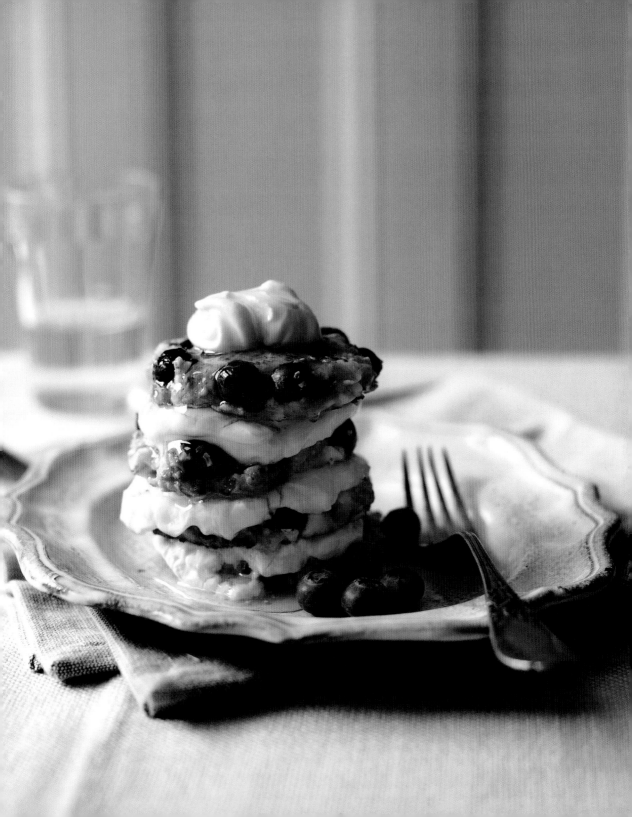

Fruity Yogurt Crunch >

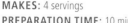

MAKES: 4 servings
PREPARATION TIME: 10 minutes
COOKING TIME: 2 minutes

15g/½oz whole almonds
15g/½oz sunflower seeds
600g/1lb 5oz/heaped 2⅓ cups
 reduced-fat Greek yogurt
200g/7oz watermelon, skin removed,
 deseeded and cut into bite-sized
 pieces
150g/5½oz blackberries or blueberries
4 tsp agave syrup

1 Heat a non-stick frying pan over a low heat. Dry-fry the almonds and sunflower seeds for 2 minutes, stirring occasionally, until lightly toasted. Watch carefully so they do not burn. Remove from the heat and leave to cool completely, then roughly chop.

2 Spoon 1 tablespoon of the yogurt into a tall glass and top with a layer of watermelon and blackberries. Repeat the layers until you reach the top of the glass. Repeat with the remaining ingredients and three more glasses to make 4 equal portions. Sprinkle with the toasted almonds and sunflower seeds, drizzle with agave syrup and serve.

Nutritional analysis per serving: Calories 159kcal **Protein** 13.7g **Carbohydrates** 18.3g **Fat** 4.2g

Quinoa Porridge with Apple & Raisins

MAKES: 4 servings
PREPARATION TIME: 10 minutes
COOKING TIME: 20 minutes

200g/7oz/1 cup quinoa
625ml/21½fl oz/2½ cups skimmed
 milk or soya milk
2 red apples, 1 unpeeled, chopped
 and cored and 1 left whole
40g/1½oz/⅓ cup flame raisins
1 cinnamon stick
4 tsp agave syrup
4 tbsp chopped Brazil nuts, to serve
ground cinnamon, to serve

1 Put the quinoa and 500ml/17fl oz/2 cups of the milk in a saucepan and bring to the boil over a medium heat. Reduce the heat to low and simmer for 5–10 minutes until soft. Add the chopped apple, raisins and cinnamon stick and cook for a further 3 minutes. Remove the cinnamon stick and cook for another 2 minutes until all the liquid has been absorbed.

2 Put the remaining milk in a saucepan and warm, stirring, over a medium-low heat. Meanwhile, core and grate the whole apple. When the milk is warm, pour the quinoa mixture into bowls, making sure you have 4 equal portions. Pour warm milk over each serving, then drizzle with agave syrup and top with grated apple, Brazil nuts and a pinch of cinnamon. Serve warm.

Nutritional analysis per serving: Calories 376kcal **Protein** 14.5g **Carbohydrates** 25g **Fat** 12g

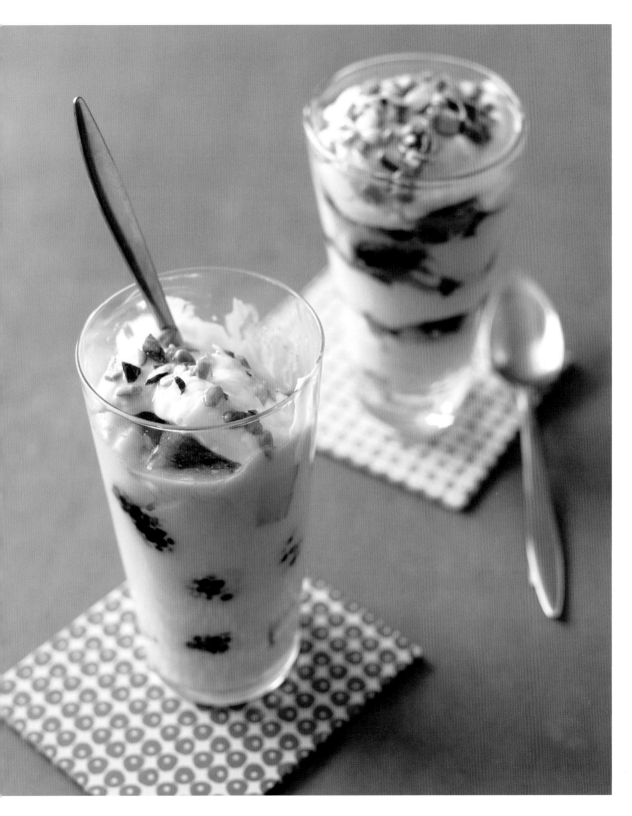

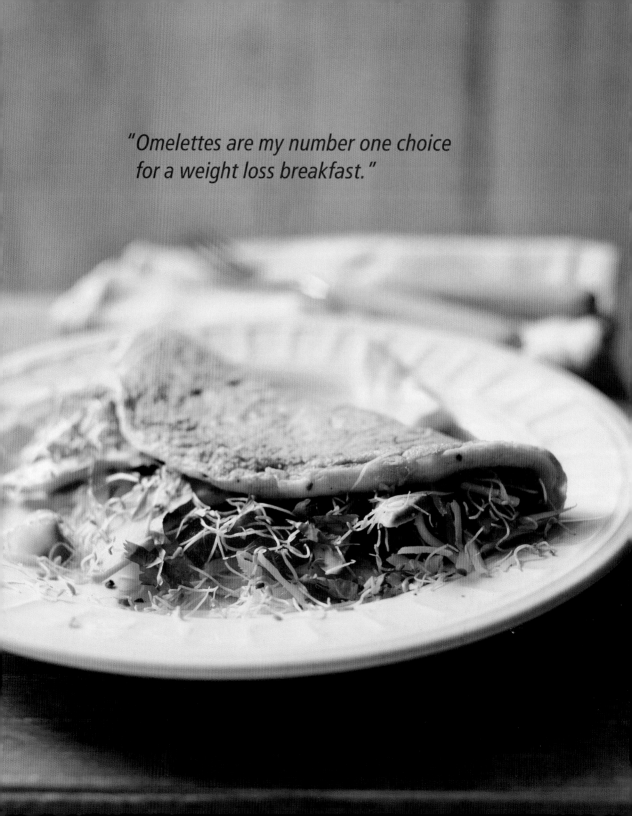

"Omelettes are my number one choice
for a weight loss breakfast."

Calfornia Superfood Omelette

MAKES: 4 servings
PREPARATION TIME: 10 minutes
COOKING TIME: 20 minutes

Omelettes are high in protein, which makes you feel full and helps you to manufacture S Factor hormones. Eggs also contain vitamin D, which is an appetite-suppressant, and the yolks contain choline which helps you feel sharp and focused. They're the perfect way to start your day.

extra virgin olive oil cooking spray
12 eggs, beaten
100g/3½oz reduced-fat mature cheese, grated
2 tomatoes, chopped
2 avocados, peeled, pitted and sliced
4 handfuls of alfalfa sprouts
1 handful of chopped coriander leaves
1 lemon, halved, plus extra wedges to serve
fine sea salt and freshly ground black pepper

1 Preheat the grill to medium-high and mist a non-stick frying pan with cooking spray. Season the eggs with salt and pepper and lightly whisk with a fork.

2 Add one-quarter of the egg mixture to the pan, shaking the pan to evenly coat the base. Put the pan under the grill for 5 minutes, occasionally pulling the edges of the mixture towards the centre of the pan, until set.

3 Slide the omelette onto a plate. Sprinkle one-quarter of the cheese, tomatoes, avocados, sprouts and coriander over the top, followed by a squeeze of lemon juice. Fold the omelette in half to enclose the fillings and cover with foil to keep warm. Repeat with the remaining egg mixture and fillings to make 3 more omelettes, misting the pan again with cooking spray if necessary. Serve hot with lemon wedges for squeezing over.

Nutritional analysis per serving: Calories 346.1kcal **Protein** 13.2g **Carbohydrates** 1.3g **Fat** 22g

Grilled Portobello Mushrooms with Roasted Vine Tomatoes

MAKES: 4 servings
PREPARATION TIME: 10 minutes
COOKING TIME: 16 minutes

A cooked breakfast doesn't have to be a fat attack. Taking the vegetarian route, and oven baking instead of frying the mushrooms, cuts your potential for gaining extra flubber. Feta is made from sheep's milk not cow's milk, and my clients have found this causes less bloating.

500g/1lb 2oz cherry vine tomatoes
1 tbsp balsamic vinegar
extra virgin olive oil cooking spray
2 tbsp extra virgin olive oil
juice of 1 lemon
2 tbsp chopped chives, plus 1 tbsp
  extra to serve
8 large Portobello mushrooms, stalks
  discarded
200g/7oz feta cheese
freshly ground black pepper

1 Preheat the oven to 180°C/350°F/Gas 4 and line a baking tray with foil. Put the tomatoes on the tray and evenly sprinkle the balsamic vinegar over the top. Mist the tomatoes with cooking spray and season with pepper. Bake for 10 minutes until the tomatoes start to collapse, then remove from the oven.

2 Meanwhile, make the marinade for the mushrooms. Mix together the olive oil, lemon juice and chives in a bowl. Preheat the grill to medium-high. Brush the marinade over the mushrooms, reserving any remaining marinade.

3 Mist a non-stick, ovenproof frying pan with cooking spray and heat over a medium heat. Add the mushrooms, cap-side up, and cook for 3 minutes, then turn over. Crumble the feta over the gills and drizzle with the reserved marinade. Put the pan under the grill for 2–3 minutes until the cheese bubbles. Spoon any pan juices over the top of each mushroom and sprinkle with chives. Divide the mushrooms and tomatoes into 4 equal portions and serve.

Nutritional analysis per serving: Calories 180kcal Protein 9.3g Carbohydrates 6.6g Fat 11.6g

Cowboy Breakfast

Baked beans are the ultimate comfort breakfast on a cold day, and making your own means they don't have to contain sugar. The crispy bacon adds a crunchy, salty contrast to the sweet tomato sauce.

MAKES: 4 servings
PREPARATION TIME: 15 minutes
COOKING TIME: 1¾ hours

extra virgin olive oil cooking spray
2 onions, chopped
2 garlic cloves, chopped
1 red pepper, deseeded and finely chopped
1 tsp paprika
¼ tsp ground cloves
2 tbsp tomato purée
125ml/4fl oz/½ cup passata
1 tbsp stevia-based natural sweetener or xylitol
220g/7¾oz haricot beans, drained and rinsed
1½ tsp Worcestershire sauce
8 back bacon rashers, trimmed of fat
fine sea salt

1 Preheat the oven to 150°C/300°F/Gas 2. If using wooden skewers, soak them in cold water for at least 30 minutes before grilling.

2 Mist an ovenproof casserole dish with cooking spray and heat over a medium-high heat. Add the onions, garlic and pepper and fry for 5 minutes until softened. Sprinkle over the paprika and cloves and cook for 1 minute, then add the tomato purée, passata, natural sweetener and 150ml/5floz/scant ⅔ cup water and bring to the boil over a high heat. Reduce the heat to low and simmer for 10 minutes. Remove from the heat and leave to cool a little. Purée the vegetables with a hand blender, or transfer to a blender or food processor and process until smooth. Return the mixture to the dish, if necessary.

3 Add the beans and Worcestershire sauce to the mixture and season with salt. Return the dish to the heat and bring to the boil over a medium-high heat. Cover with a lid and bake in the oven for 1½ hours or until the beans are tender, but not completely soft.

4 Ten minutes before the end of the cooking time, preheat the grill to medium-high. Thread 2 rashers of bacon onto each of four skewers, gathering the rashers until they appear slightly ruched. Cook for 5 minutes on each side until crisp, then carefully remove the skewers. Divide the beans and bacon into 4 equal portions and serve.

Nutritional analysis per serving: Calories 237kcal **Protein** 25g **Carbohydrates** 18.6g **Fat** 7.2g

Buckwheat Blinis with Smoked Salmon & Lemon Crème Fraîche

MAKES: 4 servings
PREPARATION TIME: 25 minutes, plus 10 minutes standing
COOKING TIME: 15 minutes

Despite the name, buckwheat is actually a low GI seed, not a grain. This breakfast is a good way to ease "carb belly" – the bloating you can experience after eating too much wheat flour.

200ml/7fl oz/scant 1 cup skimmed milk or soya milk
½ tsp dried active yeast
½ tsp caster sugar
1 egg, separated
75g/2½oz/heaped ½ cup buckwheat flour
75g/2½oz/½ cup wholemeal flour
a pinch of fine sea salt
extra virgin olive oil cooking spray
200g/7oz smoked salmon

FOR THE CRÈME FRAÎCHE:
a squeeze of lemon juice
150g/5½oz/scant ⅔ cup reduced-fat crème fraîche
2 tbsp chopped dill, plus 1 tbsp extra to serve

1 To make the blini batter, pour the milk into a saucepan and heat gently over a low heat until lukewarm – take care not to let it become too hot or the yeast will die. Remove the pan from the heat. Add the yeast and sugar and leave to stand, covered, in a warm place for 10 minutes, until the mixture starts to froth.

2 Add the egg yolk to the yeast mixture and whisk until combined. Sift the flours and salt into a mixing bowl. Make a well in the centre of the flour mixture and gradually whisk in the yeast mixture to make a thick batter. In a clean bowl, whisk the egg white until it forms soft peaks, then fold into the batter, using a metal spoon.

3 To make the crème fraîche, put the lemon juice, crème fraîche and dill in a small bowl and stir until combined. Cover and leave to chill in the fridge until needed.

4 Preheat the oven to 100°C/200°F/Gas ½. Mist a non-stick frying pan with cooking spray and heat over a medium heat. Working in batches, pour 1 tablespoon of the batter into the pan to make a blini and repeat, spacing the blinis slightly apart. Cook for 2–3 minutes on each side until the tops bubble. Keep warm in the oven while you repeat with the remaining batter to make 12 blinis, misting the pan again with cooking spray if necessary. Spread 1 teaspoon of lemon crème fraîche over each each blini, then top with smoked salmon. Divide into 4 equal portions, sprinkle with dill and serve.

Nutritional analysis per serving: Calories 223kcal **Protein** 16.9g **Carbohydrates** 17.5g **Fat** 9.2g

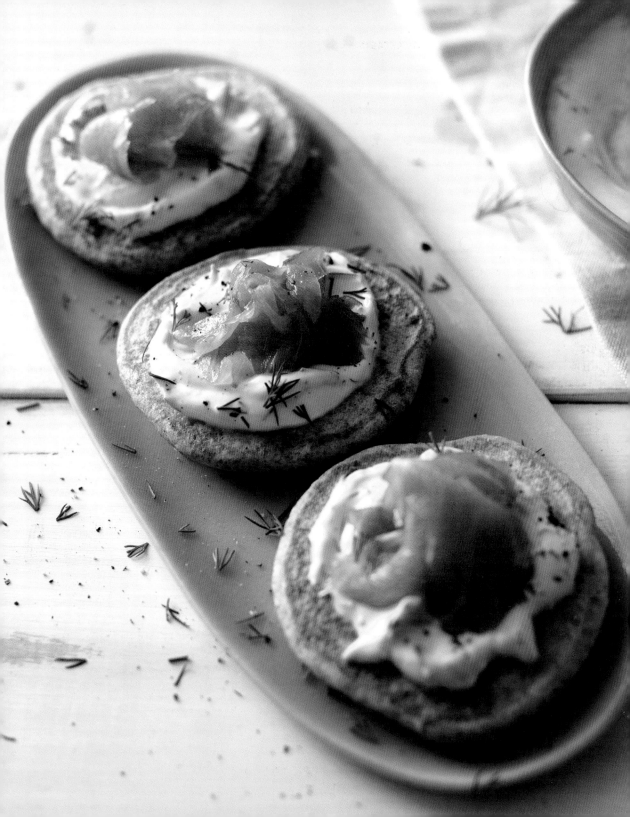

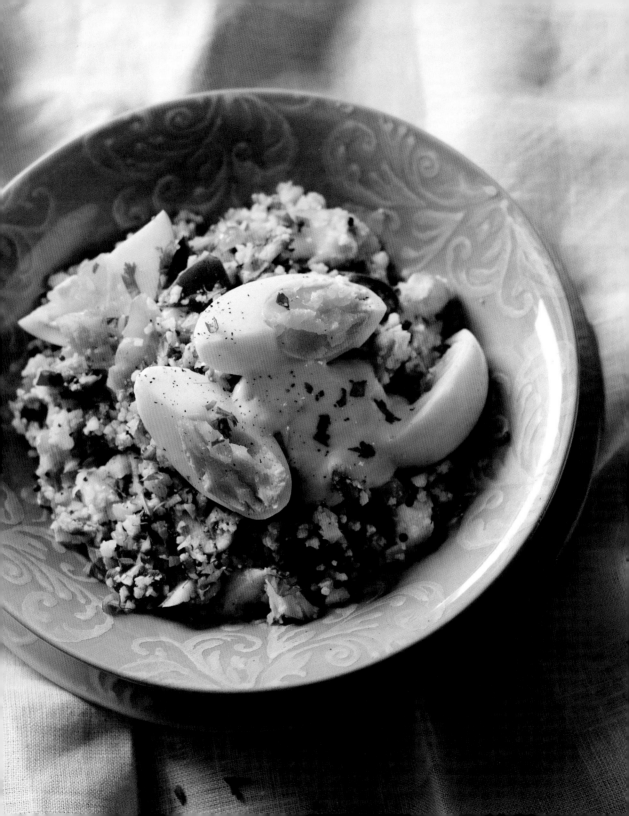

Smoked Haddock Vedgerie

MAKES: 4 servings
PREPARATION TIME: 20 minutes
COOKING TIME: 25 minutes

Kedgeree usually calls for mountains of white rice. This version still has brain-friendly haddock but uses cauliflower instead of rice, which lightens the whole dish.

4 eggs
4 undyed smoked haddock fillets, each about 120g/4¼oz
2 bay leaves
1 head of cauliflower, broken into florets
extra virgin olive oil cooking spray
2 onions, chopped
2 garlic cloves, peeled
1.5cm/⅝in piece of root ginger, peeled and grated
400g/14oz button mushrooms, sliced
1 tbsp mild curry powder
4 tsp black mustard seeds
4 tomatoes, chopped
juice of 1 lemon
1 handful of chopped coriander leaves, plus 1 tbsp extra to serve
1 red chilli, deseeded and chopped
4 tbsp reduced-fat natural yogurt
freshly ground black pepper (optional)

1 Bring a saucepan of water to the boil and add the eggs. Return to the boil and cook for 8 minutes. Remove the eggs from the pan and rinse under cold running water for 1 minute to stop them from cooking any further. Leave to one side until cool enough to handle, then peel and quarter.

2 Meanwhile, put the haddock and bay leaves in a clean saucepan. Add enough water to just cover and bring to the boil over a medium-high heat. Reduce the heat to low and simmer, covered, for 5 minutes until the fish is cooked through and opaque. Remove from the heat and drain the haddock, discarding the bay leaves. When the haddock is cool enough to handle, flake the fish, discarding the skin and any bones. Wrap in foil and leave to one side.

3 Put the cauliflower in a food processor and process until it resembles rice grains. Transfer to a steamer, or to a colander over a pan filled with about 5cm/2in water and bring to the boil. Cover and steam for 4 minutes until al dente.

4 Mist a non-stick frying pan with cooking spray and heat over a medium-high heat. Add the onions, garlic and ginger and cook for 5 minutes until softened. Add the mushrooms, curry powder and mustard seeds and cook, stirring, for a further 5 minutes, adding 1 tablespoon water to prevent the mixture from sticking to the bottom of the pan, if necessary.

5 Add the tomatoes and lemon juice and stir until combined. Remove from the heat and stir in the haddock, cauliflower rice, coriander and chilli. Divide the vedgerie into 4 equal portions, then top with yogurt and sprinkle with coriander. Serve with the hard-boiled eggs, and with a little black pepper, if you like.

Nutritional analysis per serving: Calories 249.3kcal **Protein** 35.2g **Carbohydrates** 146.4g **Fat** 8.5g

Chicken with Puy Lentils

MAKES: 4 servings
PREPARATION TIME: 15 minutes
COOKING TIME: 25 minutes

Lentils are a brilliant source of fibre. However, they're also 75 per cent carbs, so it pays to combine them with a lean protein like chicken to balance your S Factor hormones and achieve speedy weight loss.

extra virgin olive oil cooking spray
4 boneless, skinless chicken breasts, each about 120g/4¼oz
2 garlic cloves, chopped
750ml/26fl oz/3 cups low-sodium chicken stock
finely grated zest and juice of 1 lemon
200g/7oz/1 cup puy lentils
200g/7oz cherry vine tomatoes
1 handful of finely chopped parsley leaves, plus 1 tbsp extra to serve
fine sea salt and freshly ground black pepper

1 Mist a non-stick frying pan with cooking spray and heat over a medium-high heat. Add the chicken and cook for 2–3 minutes on each side until browned. Add the garlic and cook for a further 2 minutes.

2 Preheat the oven to 180°C/350°F/Gas 4. Pour in 250ml/9fl oz/1 cup of the stock and stir in the lemon zest and juice. Simmer for 10–15 minutes until the chicken is cooked through and the juices run clear when the thickest part of the meat is pierced with the tip of a sharp knife or skewer. Remove the pan from the heat. Transfer the chicken to a plate, cover with foil and leave to rest for at least 5 minutes, then slice. Reserve any remaining pan juices.

3 Meanwhile, pour the lentils and the remaining stock into a saucepan. Bring to the boil over a medium-high heat, then reduce the heat to low and simmer for 20 minutes until the lentils are tender and cooked through. Put the vine tomatoes on a baking tray, mist with cooking spray and season lightly with salt and pepper. Roast in the oven for 10–15 minutes.

4 When the lentils are cooked, drain well and stir in the parsley. Divide into 4 equal portions and top with the chicken slices. Spoon over any remaining pan juices, sprinkle with parsley and serve with the roasted vine tomatoes.

Nutritional analysis per serving: Calories 280.5kcal **Protein** 30.5g **Carbohydrates** 26.6g **Fat** 14.3g

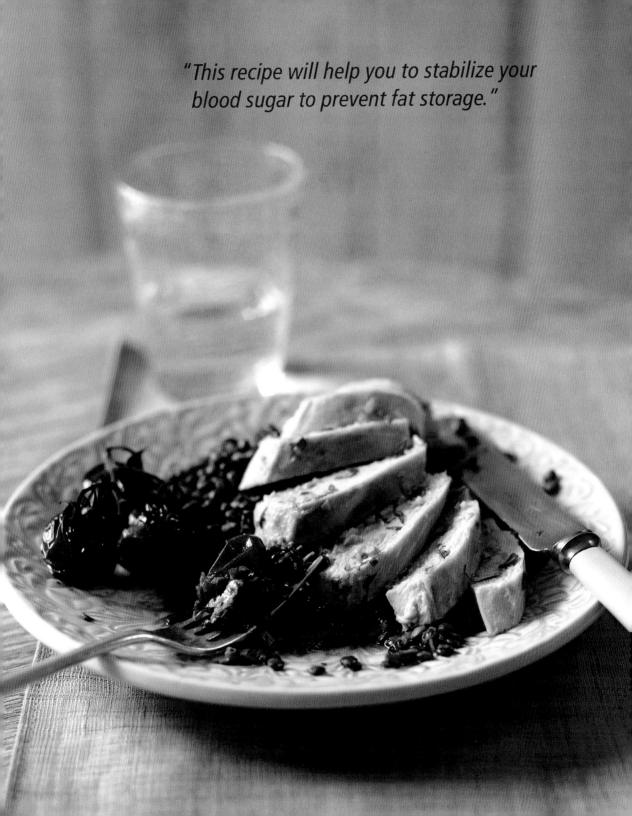

"This recipe will help you to stabilize your blood sugar to prevent fat storage."

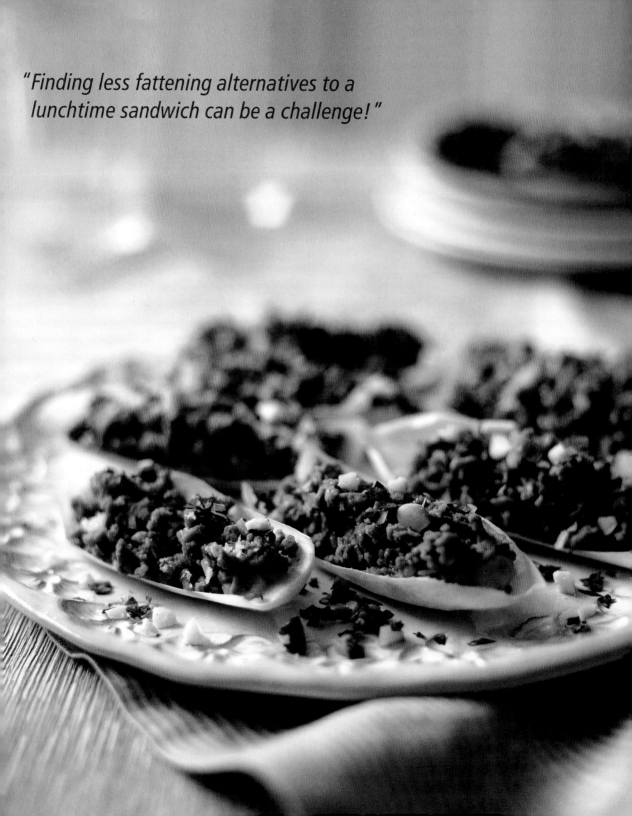

"*Finding less fattening alternatives to a lunchtime sandwich can be a challenge!*"

S ○ Cantonese Pork in Chicory
D A Spoons

MAKES: 4 servings
PREPARATION TIME: 10 minutes
COOKING TIME: 20 minutes

Forget boring, stodgy sandwiches, this lunch recipe uses chicory leaves (which have a natural spoon shape) to hold the filling. The slight bitterness of the chicory contrasts nicely with the sweet and delicious pork.

500g/1lb 2oz pork mince
2 tbsp dark soy sauce
3 tbsp oyster sauce
1 tsp stevia-based natural sweetener
   or xylitol
1 tsp sesame oil
a pinch of freshly ground black pepper
extra virgin olive oil cooking spray
2 garlic cloves, finely chopped
100g/3½oz tinned water chestnuts,
   drained, rinsed and finely chopped
24 chicory leaves
8 Brazil nuts, chopped, to serve
1 tbsp finely chopped coriander, to
   serve (optional)

1 Put the pork mince, soy sauce, oyster sauce, natural sweetener, sesame oil and pepper in a bowl and mix until well combined.

2 Mist a wok with cooking spray and heat over a high heat. Add the garlic and cook for 2 minutes. Add the pork mixture and cook, stirring, for 5 minutes until the pork has browned.

3 Continue cooking for 8–10 minutes until the pork is completely cooked through, adding 1 tablespoon water to prevent the pork from sticking to the bottom of the wok, if necessary. Thirty seconds before the end of the cooking time, add the water chestnuts and stir until heated through.

4 Spoon the pork mixture onto the chicory leaves and sprinkle with Brazil nuts, and with coriander, if you like. Divide into 4 equal portions and serve.

Nutritional analysis per serving: Calories 289kcal **Protein** 30.5g **Carbohydrates** 9.5g **Fat** 13.1g

Mini Feta-Stuffed Lamb Burgers with Polenta Muffins

MAKES: 4 servings
PREPARATION TIME: 15 minutes, plus 20 minutes chilling
COOKING TIME: 35 minutes

Who doesn't want a burger for lunch? By stuffing these home-made burgers with beetroot, you reduce the fat content. The flavours go really well together, too – the feta adds a spike of sharpness next to the earthy beetroot. Polenta has a much lower GI value than wheat, so it's a great alternative to the classic bun.

FOR THE BURGERS:

400g/14oz lamb mince
200g/7oz beetroot, peeled and grated
1 egg, beaten
2 tbsp chopped mint, plus 4 tsp extra to serve
1 garlic clove, crushed
75g/2½oz feta cheese, cut into four cubes
fine sea salt and freshly ground black pepper
2 large tomatoes, each cut into 4 slices, to serve

FOR THE MUFFINS:

extra virgin olive oil cooking spray
85g/3oz/heaped ½ cup polenta
1½ tsp baking powder
a pinch of fine sea salt
120g/4¼oz/scant ½ cup reduced-fat Greek yogurt, plus 4 tbsp extra to serve
1 egg, beaten
1 tbsp extra virgin olive oil
120g/4¼oz/scant ⅔ cup tinned or defrosted, frozen sweetcorn

1 To make the burgers, put the lamb mince, beetroot, egg, mint and garlic in a bowl. Season with salt and pepper and mix until well combined. Using your hands, divide the mixture into 4 equal pieces and roll each one into a ball. Press your finger into the centre of each ball to make a hollow. Stuff each hollow with a cube of feta then fold the mince mixture around the hollow to cover the cheese. Flatten the balls and shape each one into a burger. Cover and chill in the fridge for 20 minutes.

2 Meanwhile, preheat the oven to 200°C/400°F/Gas 6 and mist four holes of a deep muffin tin with cooking spray. To make the muffins, put the polenta, baking powder and salt in a large mixing bowl and mix. In a clean bowl, mix together all of the remaining ingredients. Add the yogurt mixture to the polenta mixture and beat slowly with a wooden spoon until combined.

3 Evenly spoon the mixture into the four holes of the muffin tin. Bake in the oven for 20 minutes until golden and a skewer inserted in the centre comes out clean. Remove from the oven and transfer to a wire rack to cool.

4 Heat a griddle pan over a medium heat. Cook the burgers for 6–8 minutes on each side or until they are cooked to your liking. Split the polenta muffins in half and place a slice of tomato on the bottom half of each one. Serve the burgers in the muffins, topped with another slice of tomato, yogurt and mint.

Nutritional analysis per serving: Calories 381kcal **Protein** 31g **Carbohydrates** 11.8g **Fat** 19g

Thai Hot & Sour Seafood Soup

MAKES: 4 servings
PREPARATION TIME: 30 minutes
COOKING TIME: 25 minutes

Chillies are thought to be thermogenic, which means they cause your body to burn up calories rather than storing them. This spicy soup will fire up your metabolism, and it's practically fat- and sugar-free, so you can feel virtuous come lunchtime.

250g/9oz raw unpeeled king prawns
extra virgin olive oil cooking spray
8 green chillies, halved
2cm/¾in piece of galangal or root
    ginger, peeled and grated
4 lemongrass stalks, finely chopped
    with outer leaves removed
8 dried kaffir lime leaves
1.5l/52fl oz/6 cups low-sodium
    chicken stock
125g/4½oz button mushrooms, halved
125g/4½oz baby corn, sliced
1 tbsp Thai red curry paste
500g/1lb 2oz frozen mixed cooked
    seafood, such as prawns, mussels
    and squid, defrosted
3 tbsp Thai fish sauce
juice of ½ lime
2 tbsp finely chopped coriander leaves,
    to serve
dried chilli flakes, to serve

1 Peel and devein the prawns, reserving the shells. Rinse thoroughly and leave to one side.

2 Mist a non-stick frying pan with cooking spray and heat over a high heat. Add the prawn shells and cook for 1 minute until pink. Add the chillies, galangal, lemongrass, lime leaves and stock. Bring to the boil over a high heat, then reduce the heat to low and simmer, uncovered, for 15 minutes.

3 Remove the pan from the heat and strain the stock into a clean saucepan, discarding the solids. Add the mushrooms, baby corn, uncooked prawns and curry paste and bring to the boil over a medium-high heat. Add the mixed cooked seafood, then reduce the heat to low and simmer for 3 minutes until heated through. Remove from the heat and stir in the fish sauce and lime juice. Divide into 4 equal portions, sprinkle each serving with coriander and a pinch of chilli flakes and serve.

Nutritional analysis per serving: Calories 150kcal **Protein** 27.4g **Carbohydrates** 11.8g **Fat** 2.4g

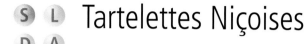

Tartelettes Niçoises

MAKES: 4 servings
PREPARATION TIME: 20 minutes, plus 10 minutes salting
COOKING TIME: 30 minutes

extra virgin olive oil cooking spray
75g/2½oz/heaped ½ cup grated courgette
20g/¾oz/2 tablespoons chickpea flour
50g/1¾oz/½ cup finely grated Parmesan cheese
1 tsp dried oregano
1 egg, beaten
1 large onion, chopped
1 garlic clove, finely chopped
400g/14oz/scant 1⅔ cups tinned chopped tomatoes
1 bay leaf
4 thyme sprigs, 1 left whole and 3 with leaves removed and chopped, plus extra sprigs to serve
1 handful of chopped parsley
a pinch of stevia-based natural sweetener or xylitol
30g/1oz drained anchovies in oil
200g/7oz tinned tuna, drained and flaked
1 handful of pitted black olives, halved
½ red onion, finely sliced
fine sea salt and freshly ground black pepper
blanched green beans, to serve

1 Preheat the oven to 200°C/400°F/Gas 6 and mist four 9cm/3½in loose-based tart tins with cooking spray. Put the courgette in a sieve, sprinkle with salt and leave to drain for 10 minutes.

2 Press down on the courgette with the back of a wooden spoon to remove as much water as possible, then transfer to a large mixing bowl. Stir in the flour, Parmesan and oregano and season with salt and pepper. Add the egg and mix thoroughly until the mixture comes together to form a "dough".

3 Divide the dough into 4 equal pieces. Using the back of a metal spoon, gently press the dough into the bottom (not the sides) of the tins and blind bake for 10 minutes until golden at the edges. Remove from the oven and set aside.

4 Meanwhile, mist a non-stick frying pan with cooking spray and heat over a medium-high heat. Add the onion and cook for 5 minutes until softened. Add the garlic, season with salt and pepper and cook for 2 minutes, adding 1 tablespoon water to prevent the onion and garlic from browning, if necessary. Stir in the chopped tomatoes, bay leaf, thyme sprig, parsley and natural sweetener. Bring to the boil over a high heat, then reduce the heat to low and simmer, uncovered, for 20 minutes until the sauce has reduced and thickened.

5 Remove the pan from the heat and discard the bay leaf and thyme sprig. Purée the sauce with a hand blender, or transfer to a blender or food processor and process until smooth. Blot the anchovies on kitchen paper, then cut each fillet in half. Spread a layer of sauce over each tartlet base, then sprinkle one-quarter of the tuna, olives, red onion, thyme leaves and anchovies over the top of each one. (Any remaining sauce can be stored in an airtight container in the fridge for up to 1 day.) Bake for 10 minutes until the base has browned and the filling has heated through. Serve one tartlet per person with a pile of crisp blanched green beans and thyme sprigs.

Nutritional analysis per serving: Calories 236kcal **Protein** 26.4g **Carbohydrates** 12.2g **Fat** 38.8g

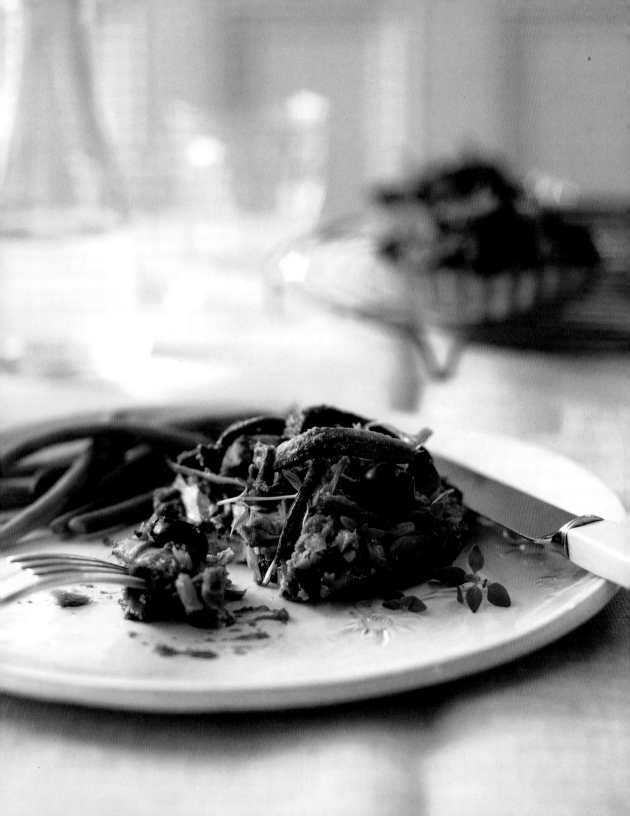

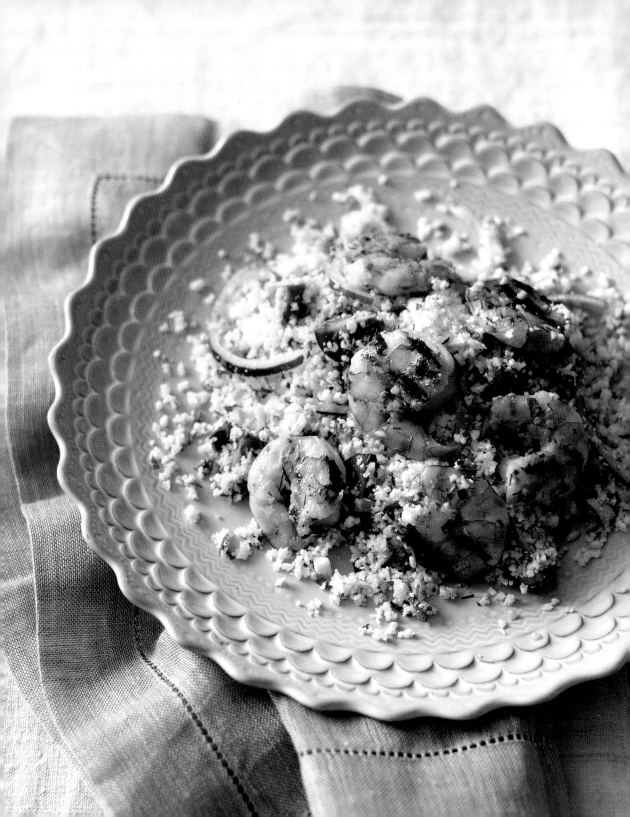

Tiger Prawns with Cauliflower "Couscous"

MAKES: 4 servings
PREPARATION TIME: 15 minutes, plus 3 hours marinating
COOKING TIME: 6 minutes

Prawns are a good source of lean protein, which is great for all your S Factor hormones, especially dopamine. By swapping normal wheat couscous for cauliflower "couscous" you immediately reduce the starch and calorie content.

400g/14oz raw tiger prawns, peeled and deveined
fine sea salt and freshly ground black pepper
lemon wedges, to serve (optional)

FOR THE MARINADE:
5 garlic cloves, crushed
2 tbsp chopped tarragon leaves
1 tbsp chopped dill
1 tbsp extra virgin olive oil

FOR THE "COUSCOUS":
1 head of cauliflower, broken into florets
1 handful of finely chopped mint leaves
1 handful of finely chopped parsley leaves, plus extra to serve
½ red onion, finely sliced
juice of ½ lemon
1 large handful of cherry tomatoes, quartered
1 tsp sweet paprika

1 If using wooden skewers, soak them in cold water for at least 30 minutes before grilling. To make the marinade, put all of the ingredients in a non-metallic bowl, season with salt and pepper and mix well. Add the prawns to the marinade and toss well, making sure the prawns are covered in the marinade. Cover and chill in the fridge for 3 hours.

2 Meanwhile, make the "couscous". Put the cauliflower in a food processor and pulse until it resembles couscous grains. Transfer to a bowl, stir in all of the remaining ingredients and season with salt and pepper. Leave to one side.

3 Use a slotted spoon to remove the prawns from the marinade, reserving the marinade. Thread about 6 prawns onto each of 4 skewers. Heat a griddle pan over a medium-high heat and cook the prawns, brushing with the reserved marinade, for about 2–3 minutes on each side until they are pink and cooked through. Remove the skewers and divide the prawns and "couscous" into 4 equal portions. Sprinkle with parsley and serve with lemon wedges for squeezing over, if you like.

Nutritional analysis per serving: Calories 148kcal **Protein** 21.3g **Carbohydrates** 4.3g **Fat** 5.6g

"This dish has very few calories, but packs a punch taste-wise."

Vietnamese Mussels

MAKES: 4 servings
PREPARATION TIME: 15 minutes
COOKING TIME: 30 minutes

I have included quite a lot of Asian-inspired recipes in this book because, rather than relying on butter, cream and cheese, they use spices to lift simple, healthy ingredients. Be sure to scrub and de-beard the mussels well or they will taste gritty.

1kg/2lb 4oz mussels in their shells
600ml/21fl oz/scant 2½ cups low-sodium chicken stock
1 small green chilli, deseeded and finely chopped
1 onion, finely chopped
2 lemongrass sticks, finely chopped with outer leaves removed
2 handfuls of finely chopped Thai basil leaves or coriander leaves, plus 1 tbsp extra to serve
fine sea salt and freshly ground black pepper

1 Remove and discard the beards from the mussels and wash them in a bowl under cold running water, scrubbing to remove all traces of grit. Discard any that float or any open ones that do not close when tapped.

2 Pour the stock into a large saucepan. Add the chilli, onion, lemongrass and Thai basil and bring to the boil over a high heat. Reduce the heat to low and simmer, covered, for 15–20 minutes until the flavours have blended. Season with salt and pepper.

3 Add the mussels to the hot stock and cook, covered, for 4–5 minutes until all the mussels have opened. Discard any mussels that do not open. Divide the mussels and the broth into 4 equal portions, sprinkle with Thai basil and serve.

Nutritional analysis per serving: Calories 181kcal **Protein** 31.3g **Carbohydrates** 5.7g **Fat** 2.6g

Middle Eastern Broad Bean & Brown Rice Soup

MAKES: 4 servings
PREPARATION TIME: 10 minutes
COOKING TIME: 30 minutes

Research suggests that we feel more satisfied after eating liquidized food, like soup, than we do after eating solid food. This recipe is a great "filler-upper" – it's full of fibre, thanks to the broad beans, and really helps to balance leptin. Beans are also a good source of magnesium, which is naturally calming, so this works well for stress-eaters too.

extra virgin olive oil cooking spray
2 onions, chopped
2 celery sticks, chopped
100g/3½oz/scant ½ cup brown rice
2 sprigs of fresh thyme
450g/1lb fresh or defrosted, frozen
   broad beans
1l/35fl oz/4 cups low-sodium vegetable
   stock
fine sea salt and freshly ground black
   pepper
4 tbsp reduced-fat Greek yogurt,
   to serve
2 tbsp finely chopped mint leaves,
   to serve

1 Mist a non-stick saucepan with cooking spray and heat over a medium-high heat. Add the onions and celery and cook for 10 minutes until the onions have softened. Add the rice, thyme, beans and stock, then season with salt and pepper and stir. Bring to the boil, then reduce the heat to low and simmer for 15 minutes until the rice is cooked.

2 Remove from the heat, discard the thyme sprigs and leave to cool a little. Divide into 4 equal portions and top each serving with 1 tablespoon of yogurt. Sprinkle with mint and serve.

Nutritional analysis per serving: Calories 208kcal **Protein** 12.3g **Carbohydrates** 35g **Fat** 10.3g

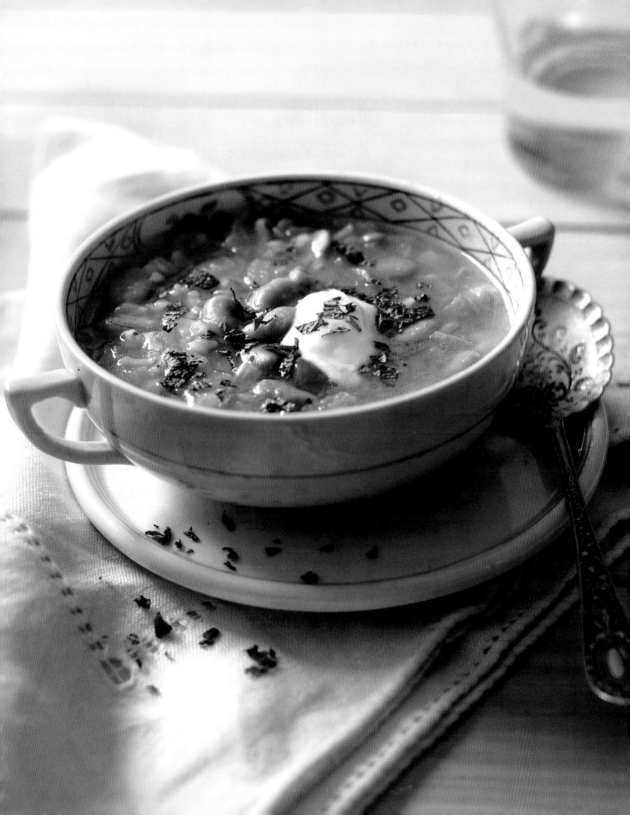

Sicilian Artichoke & Egg "Pizzas"

MAKES: 4 servings
PREPARATION TIME: 20 minutes
COOKING TIME: 45 minutes

Pizza is another food on my clients' "I really miss it" lists. However, you can make a very successful deep-pan style, soft crust base using eggs and reduced-fat cream cheese. Yes, it sounds a bit dubious, but give it a go – these Sicilian egg "pizzas" look and taste spectacular!

extra virgin olive oil cooking spray
400g/14oz reduced-fat mature Cheddar cheese, grated
230g/8¼oz/scant ½ cup reduced-fat cream cheese
2 whole eggs and 4 egg whites, beaten
1 tsp dried oregano
2 garlic cloves, crushed
4 tbsp passata
a large pinch of stevia-based natural sweetener or xylitol
4 eggs
3 bottled baby artichokes in brine, drained, patted dry and torn into pieces
1 large handful of pitted green olives
75g/2½oz/¾ cup grated Parmesan cheese
fine sea salt and freshly ground black pepper
2 grilled courgettes, halved, to serve
4 grilled red or yellow peppers, halved, to serve

1 Preheat the oven to 190°C/375°F/Gas 5 and mist four, round 9cm/3½in loose-based baking tins with cooking spray. Sprinkle one-quarter of the Cheddar over the bottom of each tin and leave to one side.

2 Beat together the cream cheese, eggs, oregano and garlic in a large mixing bowl. Evenly divide the mixture into the baking tins and smooth the surface of each one with the back of a metal spoon. Blind bake for 30 minutes until bouncy to the touch and golden brown. Remove from the oven.

3 Put the passata and natural sweetener in a small bowl. Season with salt and pepper and mix until well combined. Spread 1 tablespoon of the mixture over each pizza base. Carefully crack 1 egg into the centre of each base. Sprinkle one-quarter of the artichokes, olives and Parmesan over each base, taking care to avoid the eggs. Bake for 10–15 minutes until the egg whites are cooked through. Serve one "pizza" per person with grilled courgettes and mixed peppers.

Nutritional analysis per serving: Calories 492kcal **Protein** 46.8g **Carbohydrates** 10.3g **Fat** 31g

Moroccan Chickpea Balls with Beetroot Dip

MAKES: 4 servings
PREPARATION TIME: 30 minutes, plus cooling and 20 minutes marinating
COOKING TIME: 1 hour

FOR THE DIP:
400g/14oz beetroot
juice of ½ lemon
4 tsp extra virgin olive oil
2 tbsp finely chopped parsley leaves
400g/14oz/scant 1⅔ cups reduced-fat Greek yogurt
freshly ground black pepper

FOR THE CHICKPEA BALLS:
extra virgin olive oil cooking spray
1 onion, finely chopped
2 garlic cloves, crushed
440g/15½oz tinned chickpeas, drained and rinsed
80g/2¾oz/1 cup fresh wholemeal breadcrumbs
1 egg, beaten
a pinch of fine sea salt
2 tbsp chickpea flour, if needed
2 tbsp chermoula spice or ½ tsp harissa paste

1 Preheat the oven to 180°C/350°F/Gas 4. To make the dip, wrap the beetroot in foil and put it on a baking tray. (Leave the root attached to prevent the beetroot bleeding during cooking.) Bake for 45 minutes until a skewer inserted into the thickest part of the flesh meets no resistance. Remove from the oven and leave to cool completely.

2 Meanwhile, make the chickpea balls. Mist a non-stick frying pan with cooking spray and heat over a medium-high heat. Add the onion and garlic and fry for 5 minutes until soft. Remove from the heat and leave to cool completely.

3 Put the chickpeas in a blender or food processor and pulse until they resemble coarse breadcrumbs. Transfer to a large mixing bowl, add the onion, garlic, breadcrumbs, egg, salt and a pinch of pepper and mix well. Using your hands, divide the mixture into 12 equal pieces and roll into balls – if the mixture is too wet, stir in the flour before rolling.

4 Put the chermoula and 2 tablespoons water in a small bowl and mix together. Brush the mixture over each ball, then cover and leave to marinate in the fridge for at least 20 minutes.

5 When the beetroot is completely cool, peel and finely dice it. Transfer to a bowl and add the lemon juice, olive oil, parsley and yogurt, then season with pepper and mix well. Cover and leave to chill in the fridge until needed.

6 Mist a non-stick frying pan with cooking spray and heat over a medium-low heat. Add the chickpea balls to the pan and cook for 8–10 minutes until browned. Divide into 4 equal portions and serve with the dip.

Nutritional analysis per serving: Calories 357.6kcal **Protein** 22.3g **Carbohydrates** 48.4g **Fat** 26.2g

Courgette "Tagliatelle"

MAKES: 4 servings
PREPARATION TIME: 15 minutes
COOKING TIME: 15 minutes

Pasta, while not in itself a diet nightmare, is really hard to portion control. The recommended portion is a measly 50g/1¾oz! Another option is to make a flour-free, low GI "pasta" using vegetables. This dish uses blanched courgettes, but you could try steamed bean sprouts, stir-fried mangetout or sugar snap peas.

2 tbsp pine nuts
extra virgin olive oil cooking spray
1 red pepper, deseeded and sliced
150g/5½oz/scant 1 cup frozen peas
1 fennel bulb, thinly sliced
150ml/5fl oz/scant ⅔ cup white wine
4 courgettes
1 handful of finely chopped parsley
   leaves, plus extra to serve

1 Heat a dry frying pan until hot. Reduce the heat to medium, add the pine nuts and dry-fry for 2–3 minutes until lightly brown. (Shake the pan occasionally to ensure they do not burn.) Remove the pan from the heat, transfer the nuts to a plate and leave to one side.

2 Mist a non-stick saucepan with cooking spray and heat over a medium heat. Add the pepper and peas and cook for 4–5 minutes. Add the fennel and wine and bring up to a gentle boil, then reduce the heat to low and simmer for 5 minutes until the sauce has thickened. Remove the pan from the heat, cover with a lid and keep warm while you cook the courgette "tagliatelle".

3 Bring a large saucepan of water to the boil. Trim and halve the courgettes, then shave into ribbons, using a vegetable peeler. Plunge the courgette ribbons into the water and cook for 2 minutes until wilted and heated through. Drain well.

4 Add the courgette ribbons and parsley to the sauce and mix well. Divide into 4 equal portions, sprinkle with parsley and the toasted pine nuts and serve.

Nutritional analysis per serving: Calories 163kcal **Protein** 7.6g **Carbohydrates** 11g **Fat** 6.6g

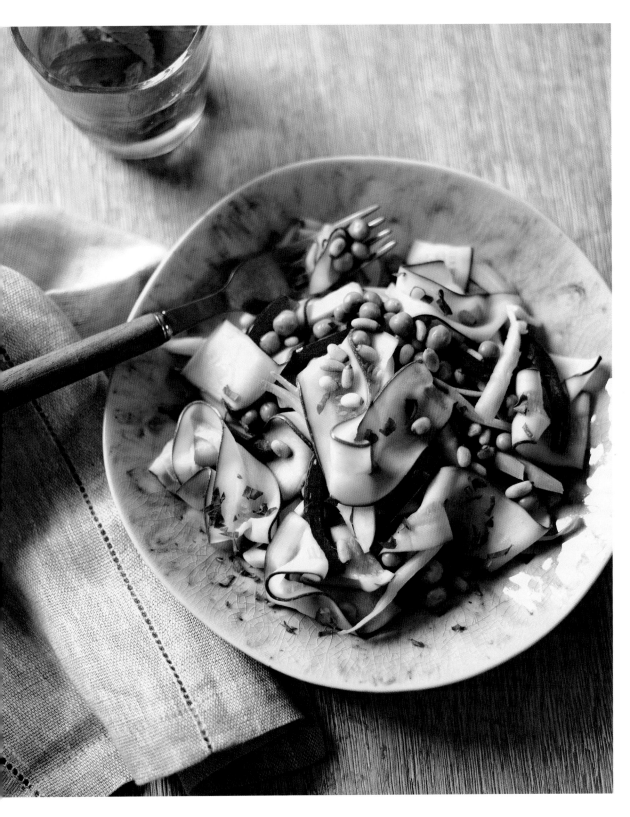

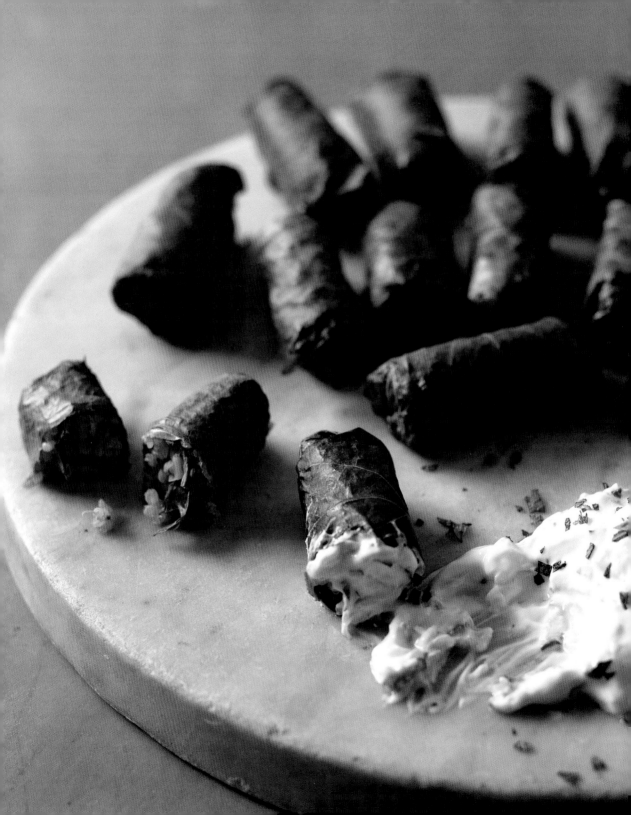

Quinoa & Pine Nut Dolmades with Tzatziki

MAKES: 4 servings
PREPARATION TIME: 20 minutes
COOKING TIME: 1 hour 10 minutes

Dolmades are made with white rice, which has little protein – so your blood sugar spikes and the sugar cravings come calling. I've put an S Factor spin on the traditional recipe by using higher protein quinoa and adding a yogurt sauce.

FOR THE DOLMADES:
extra virgin olive oil cooking spray
½ onion, chopped
1 garlic clove, crushed
250g/9oz/1¼ cups quinoa
50g/1¾oz/⅓ cup pine nuts, chopped
455ml/16fl oz/scant 2 cups low-sodium
    vegetable stock
2 tbsp finely chopped mint leaves
2 tbsp finely chopped parsley leaves
zest and juice of 1 lemon
16 bottled vine leaves or cabbage
    leaves
fine sea salt and freshly ground
    black pepper

FOR THE TZATZIKI:
½ cucumber, grated
250g/9oz/1 cup reduced-fat Greek
    yogurt
1 garlic clove, crushed
juice of ½ lemon
1 tbsp finely chopped mint leaves,
    plus extra to serve (optional)

1 To make the dolmades, mist a non-stick saucepan with cooking spray. Heat the pan over a medium-high heat, then add the onion and garlic and cook for 5 minutes until soft. Add the quinoa, pine nuts and stock and cook for a further 2 minutes. Reduce the heat to low and simmer, covered, for 15–20 minutes until the quinoa is cooked through and tender. Remove the pan from the heat. Stir in the herbs, lemon zest and juice, then season with salt and pepper and leave to cool completely.

2 Preheat the oven to 200°C/400°F/Gas 6 and mist a shallow ovenproof dish with cooking spray. Drain and rinse the vine leaves, then pat them dry with kitchen paper.

3 Spoon 1–2 teaspoons of the quinoa mixture onto the centre of 1 vine leaf. Fold the top and bottom edges over to enclose the filling, then roll up the vine leaf. Repeat with the remaining filling and vine leaves to make 16 dolmades. Transfer the dolmades to the prepared dish, packing them very tightly. Pour over 150ml/5fl oz/scant ⅔ cup boiling water. Cover with foil and bake for 40 minutes until the water has evaporated.

4 To make the tzatziki, put the cucumber in a clean kitchen towel and squeeze out as much water as possible. Transfer to a bowl, add all of the remaining ingredients and mix well. Divide the dolmades into 4 equal portions and serve with the tzatziki sprinkled with extra mint, if you like.

Nutritional analysis per serving: Calories 384kcal **Protein** 17g **Carbohydrates** 47g **Fat** 13.6g

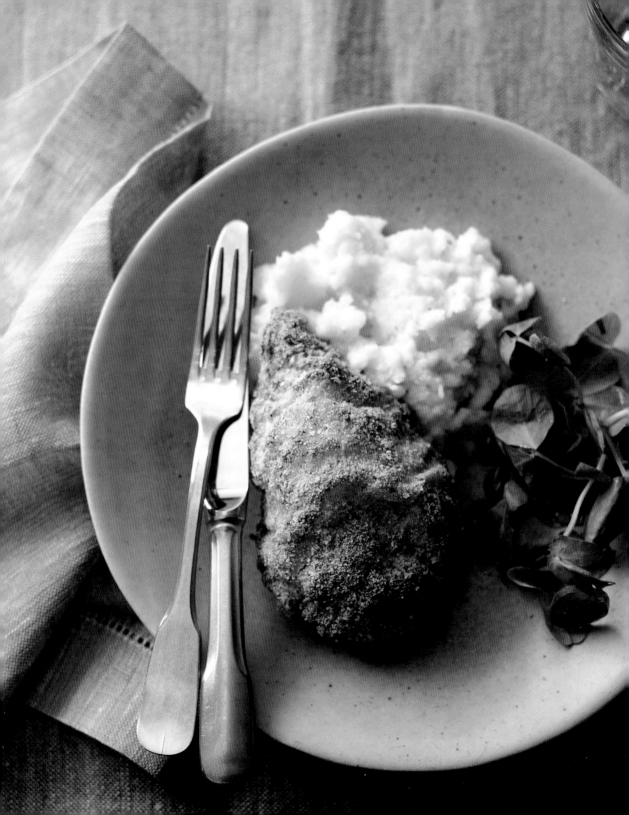

Polenta-Crusted Chicken with Cauliflower "Mash"

S L
D A

MAKES: 4 servings
PREPARATION TIME: 15 minutes
COOKING TIME: 30 minutes

Fried chicken is food for the soul, but not for the bottom – it's incredibly high in fat. My version has a healthy crust and the "mash" is practically carb free.

extra virgin olive oil cooking spray
100g/3½oz/⅔ cup polenta
50g/1¾oz/½ cup finely grated
    Parmesan cheese
1 tsp ground cayenne pepper
2 tbsp plain chickpea flour or
    soya flour
1 egg, beaten
4 boneless, skinless chicken breasts,
    each about 120g/4¼oz
fine sea salt
50g/1¾oz pea shoots, to serve

FOR THE "MASH":
1 head of cauliflower, broken into
    florets
a squeeze of lemon juice
4 tbsp reduced-fat fromage frais
freshly ground black pepper

1 Preheat the oven to 200°C/400°F/Gas 6 and mist a baking tray with cooking spray. In a bowl, mix together the polenta, Parmesan, cayenne pepper and a pinch of salt. Put the flour and egg in separate, shallow bowls. Dip each chicken breast into the flour to coat well, shaking off any excess flour, then dip each one in the egg and then in the polenta mixture.

2 Transfer the chicken to the prepared tray and bake for 20–30 minutes until the chicken is cooked through and the juices run clear when the thickest part of the meat is pierced with the tip of a sharp knife or skewer. (If the polenta starts to burn, cover with foil and continue to bake until cooked through.)

3 Fifteen minutes before serving, make the "mash". Put the cauliflower in a steamer, or in a colander over a pan with about 5cm/2in water and bring to the boil. Cover and steam for 10 minutes until very tender. Drain the cauliflower and leave to cool a little, then purée with a hand blender, or transfer to a blender or food processor and process until the mixture resembles mashed potatoes, adding water 1 teaspoon at a time until smooth, if necessary. Stir in the lemon juice and fromage frais and season with salt and pepper. Divide the "mash" and chicken into 4 equal portions and serve with pea shoots.

Nutritional analysis per serving: Calories 335kcal **Protein** 37g **Carbohydrates** 11g **Fat** 7.8g

Cretan Turkey Stew

MAKES: 4 servings
PREPARATION TIME: 15 minutes
COOKING TIME: 1 hour

Turkey is even higher in tryptophan than chicken, so it's an excellent choice for anyone wanting to balance their serotonin levels. Although it can be dry, putting turkey in a stew keeps it moist and makes a hearty dinner.

1 tbsp extra virgin olive oil
400g/14oz turkey breast, cut into chunks
2 cinnamon sticks
1 tsp cloves, crushed
1 rosemary sprig
125ml/4fl oz/½ cup gutsy red wine such as Cabernet Sauvignon
2 tbsp tomato purée
1 tsp stevia-based natural sweetener or xylitol
2 tbsp red wine vinegar
250ml/9fl oz/1 cup low-sodium chicken stock
extra virgin olive oil cooking spray
250g/9oz shallots
250g/9oz Jerusalem artichokes, scrubbed and chopped
4 courgettes
a squeeze of lemon juice
fine sea salt and freshly ground black pepper
1 tbsp finely chopped parsley leaves, to serve

1 Heat the olive oil in an ovenproof casserole dish over a medium heat. Add the turkey and cook, stirring occasionally, for 10 minutes until browned on all sides. Add the spices and rosemary and cook for a further 1 minute, then stir in the wine, tomato purée, natural sweetener, vinegar and stock. Bring to the boil over a medium-high heat, then reduce the heat to low and simmer, covered, for 25 minutes until the turkey is cooked through.

2 Mist a frying pan with cooking spray and heat over a medium-high heat. Add the shallots and artichokes and cook for 5 minutes until browned, then stir them into the turkey stew. Cook, covered, for a further 10–15 minutes until the vegetables are tender.

3 Ten minutes before the end of the cooking time, bring a large saucepan of water to the boil. Trim and halve the courgettes, then shave into ribbons, using a vegetable peeler. Plunge the courgette ribbons into the water and cook for 2 minutes until wilted and heated through, then drain well. Sprinkle with lemon juice and season with salt and pepper. Divide the courgette ribbons and stew into 4 equal portions, sprinkle with parsley and serve.

Nutritional analysis per serving: Calories 285kcal **Protein** 30.5g **Carbohydrates** 20.7g **Fat** 7.5g

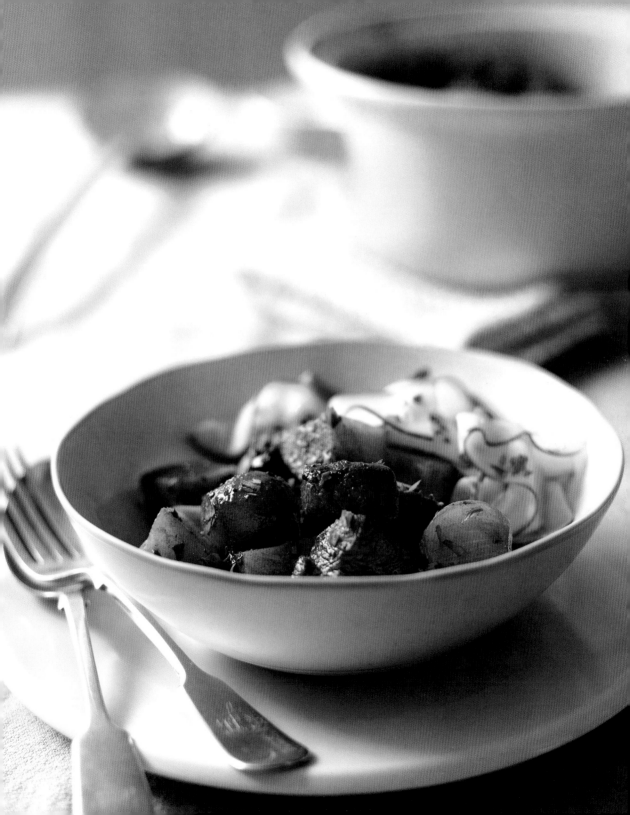

Moroccan Tagine with Broccoli & Pistachio "Tabbouleh"

MAKES: 4 servings
PREPARATION TIME: 20 minutes
COOKING TIME: 3 hours 50 minutes

This is one of my favourite dishes. Lamb is a fatty meat, but full of flavour, so mixing it with pork really adds oomph to the taste while keeping the dish healthy.

300g/10½oz lean pork shoulder, cut into chunks
300g/10½oz lamb neck, chopped
1 onion, chopped
½ garlic clove, crushed
¼ tsp cumin seeds
½ tsp coriander seeds
½ cinnamon stick
a pinch of cayenne pepper
375ml/13fl oz/1½ cups low-sodium chicken stock
2 carrots, sliced
50g/1¾oz/⅓ cup whole almonds
3 unsulphured dried apricots, halved
juice of 1½ lemons, plus the zest of ½ lemon, and extra wedges to serve
1½ tsp agave syrup
1 handful of shelled, unsalted pistachios
2 broccoli heads, broken into florets
½ red onion, finely sliced
2 handfuls of chopped parsley leaves
2 handfuls of chopped coriander leaves, plus 1 tbsp extra to serve
2 handfuls of chopped mint leaves
1 pomegranate
1 tsp extra virgin olive oil
1 tsp natural sweetener made from stevia extract or xylitol

1 Preheat the oven to 190°C/375°F/Gas 5. To make the tagine, put the pork, lamb, onion, garlic, spices and cayenne pepper in an ovenproof casserole dish. Pour in the stock, cover with a lid and transfer to the oven. Cook, covered, for 2 hours until the meat is meltingly tender. Remove the dish from the oven and stir in the carrots, almonds, dried apricots and two-thirds of the lemon juice. Return the dish to the oven and cook, covered, for a further 1½ hours. Stir in the agave syrup and cook, uncovered, for another 20 minutes.

2 Twenty minutes before the end of the cooking time, make the "tabbouleh". Heat a non-stick frying pan over a low heat. Add the pistachios and dry-fry for 2 minutes, stirring occasionally, until lightly toasted. Watch carefully so they do not burn. Remove the pan from the heat and leave to one side. Put the broccoli in a food processor and pulse until it resembles breadcrumbs. Transfer to a bowl and add the toasted pistachios, red onion and herbs. Halve the pomegranate and, holding each half over the bowl, bash the outer skin with a wooden spoon until all of the seeds fall into the bowl.

3 Put the remaining lemon juice in a bowl, then add the lemon zest, olive oil and natural sweetener and mix well. Pour this dressing over the "tabbouleh" and mix well. Remove and discard the cinnamon stick from the tagine. Divide the tagine and "tabbouleh" into 4 equal portions, sprinkle with coriander and serve with lemon wedges for squeezing over.

Nutritional analysis per serving: Calories 314kcal **Protein** 36.2g **Carbohydrates** 26g **Fat** 15.9g

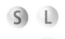

Shepherd's Pie

MAKES: 4 servings
PREPARATION TIME: 30 minutes
COOKING TIME: 1½ hours

Shepherd's pie is something many of us grew up with, but it's definitely more of a "line your ribs" than a "lose your bingo wings" dish. I've tweaked the traditional recipe by adding more veg and swapping the pure potato top for a lower GI combo of cauliflower and sweet potato.

500g/1lb 2oz sweet potatoes, chopped
500g/1lb 2oz cauliflower, broken into
   florets
2 tbsp reduced-fat fromage frais
a squeeze of lemon juice
a pinch of cayenne pepper
extra virgin olive oil cooking spray
1 onion, chopped
2 large carrots, chopped
500g/1lb 2oz lean lamb mince
2 tbsp Worcestershire sauce
2 tbsp tomato paste
1 sprig of rosemary
220ml/7½fl oz/scant 1 cup
   low-sodium lamb stock
200g/7oz/1¼ cups frozen peas
50g/1¾oz grated Parmesan cheese
fine sea salt and freshly ground
   black pepper
steamed carrots, to serve
steamed green beans, to serve

1 To make the topping, put the sweet potatoes in a large saucepan and cover with water. Bring to the boil over a medium-high heat, then reduce the heat to low and simmer for 10 minutes. Add the cauliflower, then cover with a tight-fitting lid and cook for a further 10 minutes until all of the vegetables are tender. Remove from the heat, drain well and leave to cool a little. Transfer to a blender or food processor. Add the fromage frais, lemon juice and cayenne pepper and season with salt and pepper. Process until smooth and leave to one side.

2 Preheat the oven to 190°C/375°F/Gas 5. Mist a heavy-based, ovenproof casserole dish with cooking spray and heat over a medium-high heat. Add the onion and carrots and cook for 5 minutes. Stir in the lamb mince and cook for another 5–10 minutes until browned, breaking up the meat and adding 1 tablespoon water to prevent the mixture from sticking to the bottom of the dish, if necessary.

3 Add the Worcestershire sauce, tomato paste, rosemary and stock. Bring to the boil, then reduce the heat to low and simmer for 15 minutes. Add the peas and cook for a further 5–10 minutes until the sauce has thickened.

4 Divide the filling equally into four small baking dishes. Spread one-quarter of the topping over the top of each filling. Fluff up the tops with a fork and sprinkle each one with one-quarter of the Parmesan. Bake for 20–25 minutes until the tops are crisp and golden. Serve each pie with steamed carrots and green beans.

Nutritional analysis per serving: Calories 451kcal **Protein** 31.4g **Carbohydrates** 37.6g **Fat** 11.3g

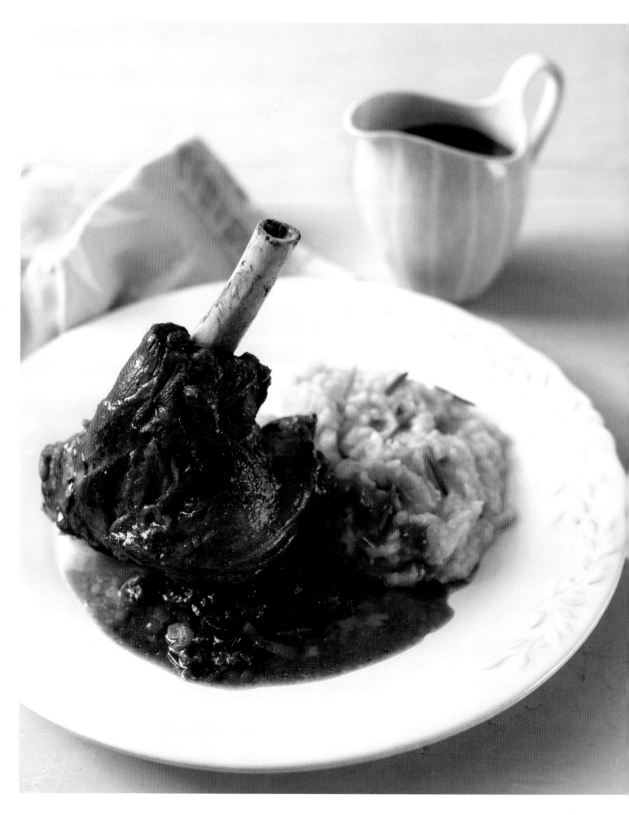

Braised Lamb Shanks with Lentil & Rosemary Mash

MAKES: 4 servings
PREPARATION TIME: 10 minutes
COOKING TIME: 2¼ hours

Lamb shanks don't have to be off the menu if you're trying to lose weight. The S Factor twist is you don't add any cream or butter to the sauce, but instead use the juices as a gravy over the high-fibre lentil mash.

FOR THE LAMB SHANKS:
extra virgin olive oil cooking spray
4 small lamb shanks, each about
    200g/7oz
1 red onion, finely sliced
1 garlic bulb, cloves peeled and sliced
2 sprigs of rosemary
400g/14oz/scant 1⅔ cups tinned
    chopped tomatoes
1 tbsp balsamic vinegar
175ml/5½fl oz/⅔ cup red wine
200ml/7fl oz/generous ¾ cup low-
    sodium lamb stock

FOR THE MASH:
200g/7oz/heaped ¾ cup yellow or
    orange lentils
1 onion, chopped
2 garlic cloves, chopped
1 rosemary sprig, plus 1 tbsp chopped
    rosemary leaves to serve
juice of ½ lemon
fine sea salt and freshly ground
    black pepper

1 Preheat the oven to 160°C/315°F/Gas 2–3 and mist an ovenproof casserole dish with cooking spray. Heat the dish over a medium-high heat and cook the lamb shanks for 5 minutes until browned all over. Remove the lamb shanks from the dish and leave to one side.

2 Add the red onion to the dish and cook for 5 minutes, adding 1 tablespoon water to prevent it from sticking, if necessary. Add the garlic and cook for a further 5 minutes until the onion has softened. Stir in all of the remaining ingredients, then return the lamb shanks to the dish. Cover with a lid, transfer to the oven and cook for 2 hours until the meat is tender and falling off the bone.

3 Thirty-five minutes before serving, make the mash. Put the lentils, onion, garlic and rosemary in a saucepan. Add enough water to just cover the ingredients and bring to the boil over a medium-high heat. Reduce the heat to low and simmer, covered, for 30 minutes until the lentils are tender. Remove from the heat and leave to cool slightly. Discard the rosemary sprig and transfer the mixture to a blender or food processor. Add the lemon juice and season with salt and pepper, then process until smooth. Divide the lamb shanks and mash into 4 equal portions. Drizzle the cooking juices from the lamb over the top, sprinkle with rosemary and serve.

Nutritional analysis per serving: Calories 521kcal **Protein** 64.6g **Carbohydrates** 29g **Fat** 32.9g

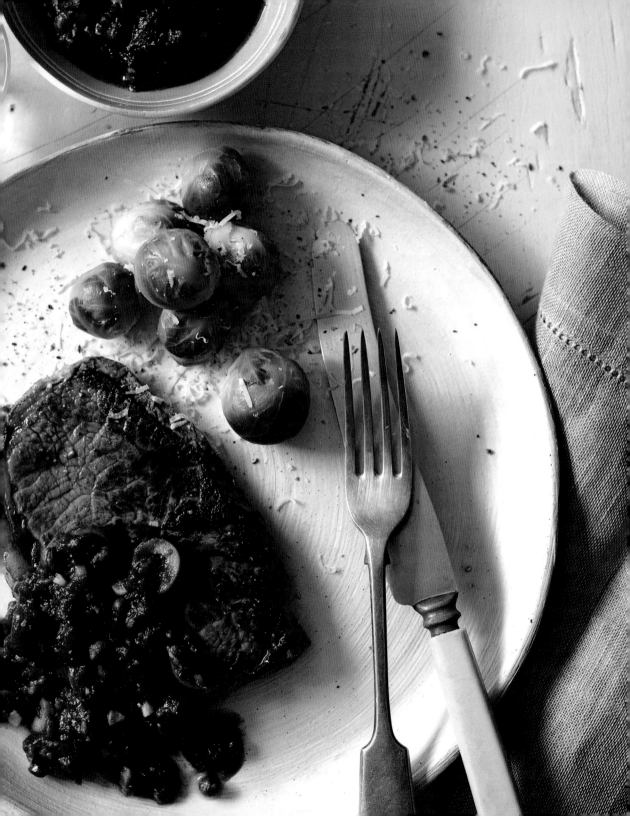

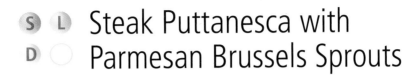

Steak Puttanesca with Parmesan Brussels Sprouts

MAKES: 4 servings
PREPARATION TIME: 15 minutes
COOKING TIME: 50 minutes

Without the familiar butter and cream-based sauces, low-fat food can get as dry as old shoe leather. Another way round this is to add a killer vegetable-based sauce like this one. Puttanesca is traditionally served over pasta, but it's fantastic with beef. I like to use it with chicken, fish and as a pizza topping, too.

extra virgin olive oil cooking spray
35g/1¼oz drained anchovies in oil
4 garlic cloves, finely sliced
1 large handful of pitted green olives, sliced
1 tbsp capers, drained and rinsed
2 tbsp dried oregano
400g/14oz/scant 1⅔ cups tinned chopped tomatoes
a pinch of stevia-based natural sweetener or xylitol
200ml/7fl oz/generous ¾ cup low-sodium beef stock
4 sirloin steaks, each about 100g/3½oz
a splash of white wine
fine sea salt and freshly ground black pepper

FOR THE BRUSSELS SPROUTS:
300g/10½oz Brussels sprouts
2 tbsp grated Parmesan cheese

1 Mist a frying pan with cooking spray and heat over a medium-high heat. Blot the anchovies on kitchen paper, then add them to the pan, followed by the garlic, olives, capers and oregano. Cook, stirring, for 5 minutes, adding 1 tablespoon water to prevent the mixture from sticking to the bottom of the pan, if necessary. Add all of the remaining ingredients, except the steaks and wine, and bring to the boil. Reduce the heat to low and simmer, covered, for 35 minutes. Remove the lid and simmer, uncovered, for a further 10 minutes until the sauce has reduced and thickened.

2 Fifteen minutes before the end of the cooking time, make the sprouts. Bring a large saucepan of water to the boil and add the sprouts. Return to the boil, then reduce the heat to a simmer and cook for 5–10 minutes until the sprouts are just tender. Drain well.

3 Meanwhile, mist a large frying pan with cooking spray and heat over a medium-high heat. Season the steaks with salt and pepper, then add them to the pan with the wine. Cook the steaks for 3–4 minutes on each side until cooked to your liking. Divide the steaks, sauce and sprouts into 4 equal portions. Evenly sprinkle the Parmesan over the top of the sprouts and serve.

Nutritional analysis per serving: Calories 389.4kcal **Protein** 63.1g **Carbohydrates** 6.9g **Fat** 17.4g

Salmon Fishcakes with Parsley Sauce & Fresh Minted Peas

MAKES: 4 servings
PREPARATION TIME: 10 minutes
COOKING TIME: 50 minutes

400g/14oz sweet potatoes, diced
extra virgin olive oil cooking spray
450g/1lb boneless, skinless salmon fillet
1 onion, sliced
1 bay leaf
570ml/20fl oz/scant 2⅓ cups skimmed
    milk or soy milk
2 spring onions, finely sliced
2 tsp chopped dill
2 tsp chopped parsley leaves
2 tsp chopped tarragon leaves
100g/3½oz/1¼ cups fresh wholemeal
    breadcrumbs
fine sea salt and freshly ground black
    pepper

FOR THE SAUCE:
170g/5¾oz/scant ¾ cup reduced-fat
    fromage frais
2 tbsp chopped parsley
30g/1oz watercress
juice and zest of ½ lemon

FOR THE PEAS:
750g/1lb 10oz fresh or defrosted,
    frozen peas
1 handful of chopped mint leaves

1 Put the sweet potatoes in a large saucepan and cover with water. Bring to the boil over a medium-high heat, then reduce the heat to low and simmer for 20 minutes. Drain well and transfer to a large bowl. Season with salt and pepper, mash until smooth and leave to one side.

2 Meanwhile, mist a large saucepan with cooking spray and heat over a medium heat. Add the salmon, onion, bay leaf and milk and season with salt and pepper. Bring to a simmer over a low heat and poach for 10 minutes until the salmon is opaque and cooked through. Remove the pan from the heat. Using a fish slice, remove the salmon from the pan and leave to cool a little.

3 Flake the salmon into the mashed potatoes. Stir in the spring onions and herbs and mix until well combined. Using your hands, divide the mixture into 8 equal pieces and shape each one into a fishcake.

4 Sprinkle the breadcrumbs onto a plate and press the fishcakes into them, making sure they are well coated in breadcrumbs. Transfer the fishcakes to a plate, then cover and chill in the fridge for 15–20 minutes.

5 Meanwhile, make the sauce and peas. Put all of the ingredients for the sauce in a food processor and process to a coarse purée. Transfer to a bowl and cover and chill in the fridge until needed. Put the peas in a saucepan and cover with water. Bring to the boil over a medium-high heat, then reduce the heat to low and simmer for 5 minutes until tender. Drain well and return to the pan. Stir in the mint, then cover with a lid and keep warm.

6 Mist a non-stick frying pan with cooking spray. Working in batches, fry the fishcakes over a medium heat for 4–6 minutes on each side until golden. Divide the fishcakes, peas and sauce into 4 equal portions and serve.

Nutritional analysis per serving: Calories 499kcal **Protein** 57.9g **Carbohydrates** 68.2g **Fat** 15.3g

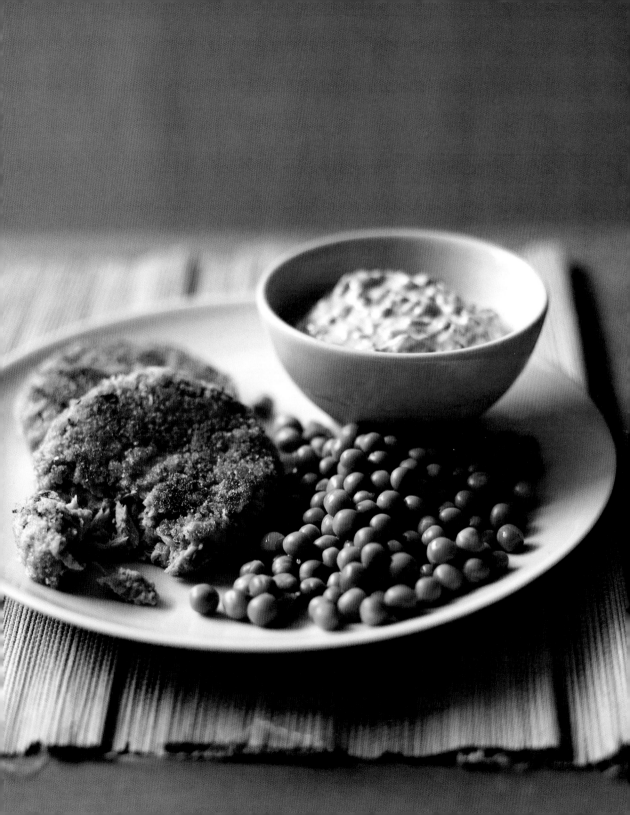

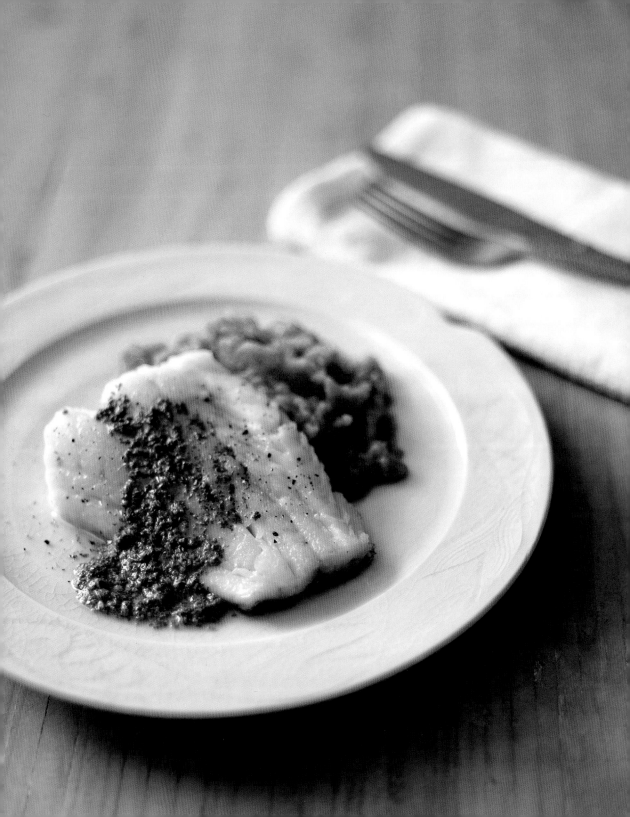

S L D A Pollock with Salsa Verde & Carrot Purée

MAKES: 4 servings
PREPARATION TIME: 20 minutes
COOKING TIME: 30 minutes

Salsa Verde is a great sauce that really lifts simple white fish and plain chicken. It's made with quite a few lugs of olive oil (healthy fat, but your thighs don't necessarily know that), so don't go dolloping it on as if there's no tomorrow. A little goes a long way to totally transform a dish.

extra virgin olive oil cooking spray
4 pollock fillets, each about 120g/4¼oz
fine sea salt and freshly ground black
  pepper

FOR THE SALSA VERDE:
115ml/3¾fl oz/scant ½ cup extra virgin
  olive oil
25g/1oz parsley leaves
1 small handful of mint leaves
leaves from 1 sprig of oregano
30g/1oz baby spinach
20g/¾oz capers, drained and rinsed
2 tsp Dijon mustard
juice of ½ lemon

FOR THE PURÉE:
1 shallot, very finely chopped
a pinch of ground ginger
300g/10½oz carrots, chopped
1 tbsp reduced-fat fromage frais
a squeeze of lemon juice

1 To make the salsa verde, put the olive oil in a blender or mini food processor. With the motor running, gradually add the herbs and spinach and blend for 1 minute. Add the capers and mustard and continue to blend until a coarse paste forms. Transfer to a bowl and stir in the lemon juice. Season with salt and pepper, then cover and leave to one side.

2 To make the purée, mist a non-stick frying pan with cooking spray and heat over a medium-high heat. Add the shallot and ginger and cook for 5 minutes. Add the carrots and 3 tablespoons water, then turn the heat down to low and cook, covered, for 15 minutes until the carrots are tender. Drain the vegetables and leave to cool a little, then purée with a hand blender, or transfer to a food processor and process until smooth. Stir in the fromage frais and lemon juice and season with salt and pepper. Cover and keep warm.

3 Mist a large, non-stick frying pan with cooking spray and heat over a medium heat. Add the pollock and cook for 4–5 minutes on each side until opaque and cooked through, adding 1 tablespoon water to stop the fish sticking to the bottom of the pan, if necessary. Season with salt and pepper. Divide the pollock and purée into 4 equal portions. Top each serving with 1 tablespoon of salsa verde and serve.

Nutritional analysis per serving: Calories 372.2kcal **Protein** 23.1g **Carbohydrates** 89g **Fat** 28.6g

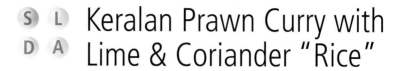

Keralan Prawn Curry with Lime & Coriander "Rice"

MAKES: 4 servings
PREPARATION TIME: 15 minutes
COOKING TIME: 20 minutes

South Indian curries are better (nutritionally) than North Indian ones because they are based around coconut milk, which contains healthy fats as opposed to ghee, which is pure sat fat. This dish goes one better and uses reduced-fat coconut milk.

1 head of cauliflower, broken into
   florets
1 tbsp chopped cashew nuts
3 red chillies, 2 deseeded and chopped
   and 1 deseeded and very finely
   chopped
finely grated zest and juice of 1 lime,
   plus 2 limes cut into wedges to serve
2 handfuls of chopped coriander leaves
1 red onion, finely chopped
5cm/2in piece of root ginger, peeled
   and grated
2 tsp coconut oil or extra virgin olive oil
2 tsp black mustard seeds
1 tsp fenugreek seeds
20 dried curry leaves
1 tsp turmeric
1 tsp black peppercorns, crushed
300ml/10½fl oz/scant 1¾ cups
   reduced-fat coconut milk
500g/1lb 2oz cooked king prawns

1 Put the cauliflower in a food processor and pulse until it resembles rice grains. Transfer to a steamer, or to a colander over a pan with about 5cm/2in water and bring to the boil. Cover and steam for 2 minutes until heated through. Transfer to a bowl and stir in the cashew nuts, the finely chopped chilli, half of the lime zest and juice and 1 handful of the coriander. Cover with foil and keep warm.

2 Put the remaining chillies, red onion, ginger and 6 tablespoons water in a blender or food processor and process until a smooth paste forms. Heat the coconut oil in a non-stick saucepan over a medium heat. Add the black mustard seeds, fenugreek seeds and curry leaves and fry for 2 minutes, then reduce the heat to low and add the chilli paste. Cook for 5 minutes until thickened, adding 1 tablespoon water to prevent the mixture from sticking to the bottom of the pan, if necessary.

3 Stir in the turmeric and peppercorns, pour in the coconut milk and bring to a simmer, stirring, over a low heat. Add the prawns and cook for 1–2 minutes until hot, then stir in the remaining lime juice and coriander. Divide the curry and cauliflower "rice" into 4 equal portions. Sprinkle with the remaining lime zest and serve with lime wedges for squeezing over.

Nutritional analysis per serving: Calories 250kcal **Protein** 26g **Carbohydrates** 10.5g **Fat** 8.6g

L D A Catalan Seafood & Fennel Stew with Courgette Purée

MAKES: 4 servings
PREPARATION TIME: 25 minutes
COOKING TIME: 35 minutes

50g/1¾oz mussels in their shells
extra virgin olive oil cooking spray
1 fennel bulb, finely sliced with the
    fronds reserved and chopped
2 leeks, finely sliced
2 garlic cloves, crushed
½ tsp paprika
2 tbsp pastis, such as Pernod
200ml/7fl oz/generous ¾ cup white wine
¼ tsp saffron
¼ tsp chopped thyme leaves
400g/14oz boneless, skinless white fish
    fillets such as pollock or hoki, cut
    into chunks
200g/7oz raw king prawns, peeled and
    deveined
200g/7oz baby octopuses, beak and
    guts removed

FOR THE PURÉE:
½ onion, finely sliced
400g/14oz courgettes, thinly sliced
60g/2¼oz/heaped ¼ cup reduced-fat
    fromage frais
a squeeze of lemon juice
fine sea salt and freshly ground black
    pepper

1   Remove and discard the beards from the mussels and wash them in a bowl under cold running water, scrubbing to remove all traces of grit. Discard any that float or any open ones that do not close when tapped.

2   Mist a large, non-stick saucepan with cooking spray and heat over a medium heat. Add the fennel, leeks and garlic and cook for 1 minute. Sprinkle in the paprika and cook for a further 8 minutes, adding 1 tablespoon water to prevent the mixture from sticking to the bottom of the pan, if necessary. Pour in the pastis and wine and bring to the boil over a medium-high heat. Cook for 5 minutes until the wine has reduced by one-third.

3   Add the mussels and cook, covered, for 5 minutes until all the mussels have opened. Discard any mussels that do not open. Transfer the mussels to a bowl, using a slotted spoon, then cover with foil and keep warm.

4   Stir the saffron and thyme into the stew and cook for 2 minutes. Add the fish, prawns and octopuses and simmer, covered, for a further 10 minutes until the fish is opaque, the prawns are pink, and the octopuses have just cooked through.

5   Meanwhile, make the purée. Mist a non-stick saucepan with cooking spray and heat over a medium-high heat. Cook the onion for 5 minutes, then add the courgettes and 100ml/3½fl oz/generous ⅓ cup water. Bring to the boil, then reduce the heat to low and simmer for 10 minutes until the courgettes are soft. Drain the vegetables and leave to cool a little, then purée with a hand blender, or transfer to a blender or food processor and process until smooth. Stir in the fromage frais and lemon juice and season with salt and pepper.

6   Return the mussels to the stew. Divide the stew and purée into 4 equal portions. Sprinkle with fennel fronds and serve.

Nutritional analysis per serving: Calories 411kcal Protein 47.5g Carbohydrates 9.3g Fat 9.4g

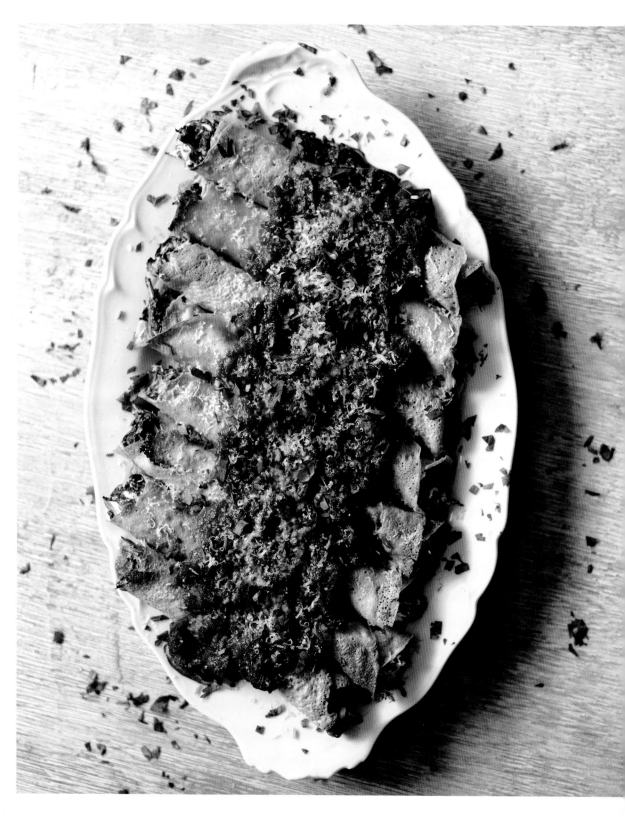

Spinach & Cheese "Cannelloni"

MAKES: 4 servings
PREPARATION TIME: 25 minutes
COOKING TIME: 1½ hours

25g/1oz/scant ¼ cup soya flour
a pinch of fine sea salt
25g/1oz/¼ cup ground almonds
3 eggs, beaten
50ml/1½fl oz/3 tbsp skimmed milk
    or soya milk
extra virgin olive oil cooking spray
400g/14oz defrosted, frozen spinach
100g/3½oz/heaped ⅓ cup reduced-fat
    ricotta cheese
100g/3½oz/heaped ⅓ cup reduced-fat
    cream cheese
a pinch of freshly grated nutmeg
2 tbsp finely grated Parmesan cheese,
    to serve
grilled courgettes, to serve

FOR THE TOMATO SAUCE:
1 garlic clove, chopped
¼ carrot, grated
2 handfuls of finely chopped parsley
    leaves, reserving 1 tbsp to serve
¼ celery stick, chopped
200g/7oz/1 cup tinned chopped
    tomatoes
1 handful of basil leaves

1 Sift the flour and salt into a mixing bowl and stir in the ground almonds. Add the eggs and milk and beat together to make a smooth batter.

2 Mist a non-stick frying pan with cooking spray and heat over a medium-high heat until hot. Working in batches, pour 3 tablespoons of the batter into the pan to make a crêpe, tilting the pan to make sure the batter evenly covers the base. Cook for 1–2 minutes on each side until golden. Transfer to a plate and repeat with the remaining batter to make 8 crêpes, misting the pan again with cooking spray before cooking each crêpe. Stack the crêpes on the plate and cover with foil to keep warm.

3 To make the tomato sauce, mist a non-stick saucepan with cooking spray. Heat over a medium-high heat and cook the garlic for 1 minute. Add the carrot, parsley and celery and cook for a further 3 minutes, adding 1 tablespoon water to prevent the mixture from sticking to the bottom of the pan, if necessary. Add the chopped tomatoes, basil and 100ml/3½fl oz/ generous ⅓ cup water and bring to the boil, then reduce the heat to low and simmer, covered, for 10 minutes. Remove the lid and simmer for a further 10 minutes until the sauce has reduced and thickened. Remove the pan from the heat and leave to one side.

4 Preheat the oven to 190°C/375°F/Gas 5 and mist a baking dish with cooking spray. Using your hands, squeeze out as much water from the spinach leaves as possible, then finely chop them. Put the ricotta, cream cheese and nutmeg in a bowl and stir until combined.

5 Spoon one-eighth of the ricotta mixture and spinach near the edge of a crêpe, then carefully roll it up into a tube. Repeat with the remaining crêpes and filling. Transfer the crêpes to the prepared dish and top with the tomato sauce, then sprinkle 1 tablespoon of the Parmesan over the top. Bake for 20–30 minutes until golden brown and bubbling. Sprinkle the remaining Parmesan and parsley over the top and divide into 4 equal portions. Serve with grilled courgettes.

Nutritional analysis per serving: Calories 264kcal **Protein** 16.7g **Carbohydrates** 12.9g **Fat** 10.4g

Fig & Feta Tart

MAKES: 4 servings
PREPARATION TIME: 10 minutes
COOKING TIME: 40 minutes

This tart has an ingenious carrot pastry base – it isn't quite as crisp as normal pastry, but it's a very pretty colour and its slightly sweet flavour is especially good with the salty feta topping. Vegetarians can skip the prosciutto.

extra virgin olive oil cooking spray
4 slices of prosciutto, trimmed of fat (optional)
50g/1¾oz feta cheese, crumbled
4 figs, quartered
1 tsp finely chopped thyme leaves, plus extra sprigs to serve
fine sea salt and freshly ground black pepper
steamed broccoli, to serve
steamed leeks, to serve

FOR THE PASTRY:
75g/2½oz/scant ½ cup grated carrot
2 tablespoons chickpea flour, sifted
50g/1¾oz/½ cup grated Parmesan cheese
a pinch of paprika
4 eggs, beaten

1 Preheat the oven to 200°C/400°F/Gas 6 and mist a loose-based, 20cm/8in fluted tart tin with cooking spray. To make the pastry, put the carrot, flour, Parmesan and paprika in a bowl and season with salt and pepper. Stir in the eggs and mix thoroughly until the mixture comes together to form a "dough". Press the dough into the bottom of the tin (not the sides) and blind bake for 20 minutes until crisp at the edges.

2 Remove the tart tin from the oven and mist the top of the pastry with cooking spray. Arrange the proscuitto, feta and figs over the top of the pastry. Sprinkle over the thyme and season with salt and pepper. Bake for 20 minutes until the cheese has melted and the proscuitto is crisp. Sprinkle with thyme sprigs and cut into 4 equal slices. Serve with steamed broccoli and leeks.

Nutritional analysis per serving: Calories 307kcal **Protein** 22g **Carbohydrates** 14g **Fat** 14.3g

"Regular pastry is a fat and flour nightmare, but this tart base is made from grated carrot, chickpea flour and eggs."

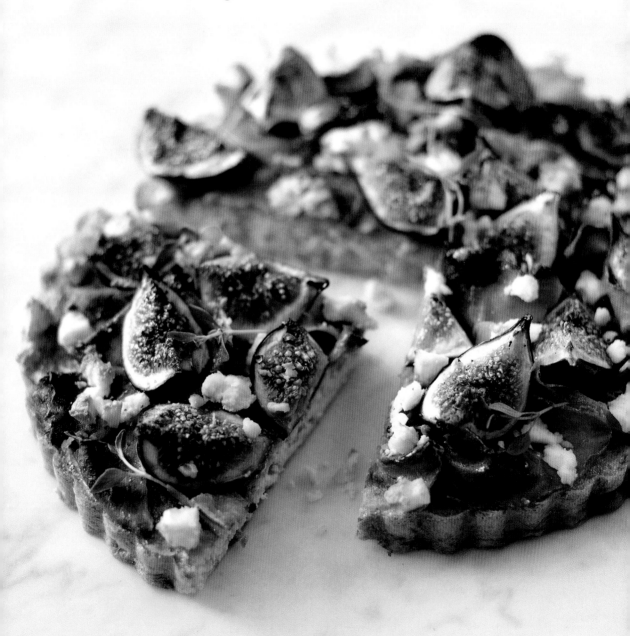

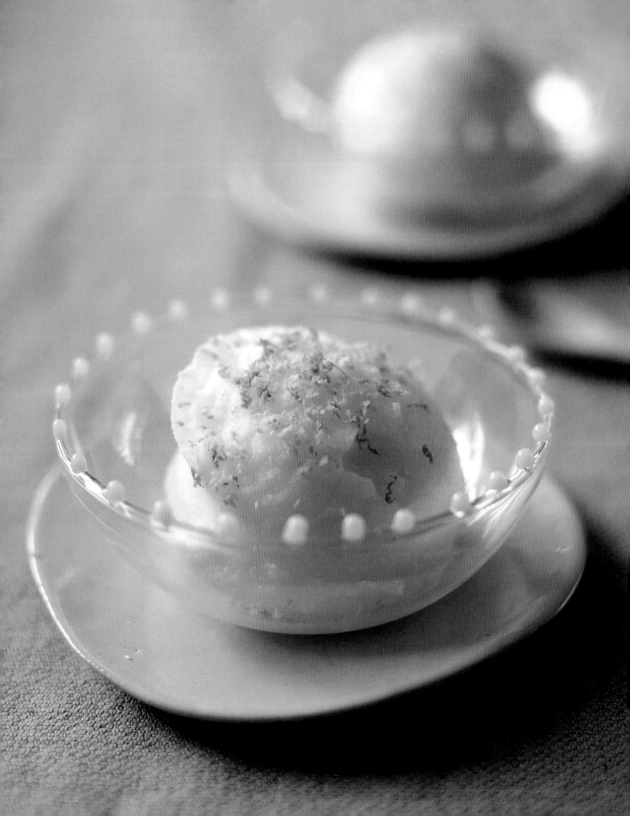

< Coconut Sorbet

MAKES: 4 servings
PREPARATION TIME: 15 minutes, plus cooling and 3 hours freezing
COOKING TIME: 5 minutes

120g/4¼oz/scant ⅔ cup stevia-based natural sweetener or xylitol
80ml/2½fl oz/⅓ cup coconut milk
a squeeze of lime juice, plus 1 tbsp lime zest to serve
35g/1¼oz/heaped ⅓ cup grated fresh or desiccated coconut

1 Put the natural sweetener and 150ml/5fl oz/scant ⅔ cup water in a saucepan. Heat over a low heat and stir until the sweetener has dissolved and the mixture is syrupy. Remove from the heat and stir in the coconut milk, lime juice and three-quarters of the coconut. Leave to cool completely. Dry-fry the remaining coconut over a medium-high heat, stirring, until toasted. Leave to one side.

2 Transfer the mixture to a freezer-proof container, and freeze, covered, for 1 hour. Transfer to a blender and process to break up any ice crystals. Return to the container and freeze, covered, for 2 hours until completely frozen. Remove from the freezer and leave to soften slightly for 5 minutes at room temperature. Divide into 4 equal portions, sprinkle with lime zest and toasted coconut and serve.

Nutritional analysis per serving: Calories 72kcal **Protein** 19.6g **Carbohydrates** 6.2g **Fat** 27g

Raspberry Granita

MAKES: 4 servings
PREPARATION TIME: 15 minutes, plus 3 hours freezing and 20 minutes standing
COOKING TIME: 5 minutes

60g/2¼ oz/scant ⅓ cup stevia-based natural sweetener or xylitol
350g/12oz raspberries
mint leaves, to serve

1 Put a fork and a freezer-proof container in the freezer. Put the natural sweetener and 250ml/9fl oz/1 cup water in a saucepan. Heat, stirring, over a low heat until the mixture is syrupy. Remove from the heat and leave to cool. Put the raspberries in a blender and process to a coarse purée. Using the back of a spoon, press the purée through a sieve into a bowl. Discard the seeds. Return the raspberry mixture to the blender, add the sweetener syrup and process until smooth.

2 Pour the mixture into the chilled container. Freeze, uncovered, for 30 minutes until ice crystals form. Scrape the granita with the chilled fork to break up any lumps and return to the freezer. Scrape the granita every 30 minutes until completely frozen, this will take about 3 hours. Remove from the freezer and leave to soften slightly for about 20 minutes at room temperature. Divide into 4 equal portions, sprinkle with mint leaves and serve.

Nutritional analysis per serving: Calories 23kcal **Protein** 4.9g **Carbohydrates** 16g **Fat** 1.4g

Champagne Jellies >

MAKES: 4 servings
PREPARATION TIME: 10 minutes
COOKING TIME: 10 minutes,
plus cooling and at least 5 hours chilling

4 tbsp stevia-based natural sweetener
    or xylitol
350ml/12fl oz/scant 1½ cups pink
    champagne or sparkling wine
6 gelatine leaves
100g/3½oz redcurrants, removed
    from the stem, or other soft fruit
    such as blackberries or raspberries
1 sheet of edible gold leaf (optional)

1 Put the natural sweetener and 100ml/3½fl oz/generous ⅓ cup hot water in a saucepan. Heat over a low heat and stir until the mixture is syrupy. Pour the champagne into a bowl, add the gelatine and leave to soak for 5 minutes. Squeeze the gelatine to return as much champagne as possible to the bowl. Add the gelatine to the syrup and whisk until dissolved, then pour the mixture into champagne and whisk until combined. Leave to cool completely. Cover with cling film and chill in the fridge for at least 1 hour until thickened.

2 Stir in the redcurrants, then pour the mixture into four glasses. Cover with cling film and leave to chill in the fridge for 4–6 hours until completely set. Decorate the jellies with pieces of gold leaf, if you like, and serve immediately.

Nutritional analysis per serving: Calories 81kcal **Protein** 11g **Carbohydrates** 5.6g **Fat** 0g

Japanese Fruit Salad

MAKES: 4 servings
PREPARATION TIME: 15 minutes,
plus cooling and 40 minutes chilling

1 green tea bag
juice of 1 lime
2 tbsp agave syrup
2 tbsp mirin or dry sherry
2 kiwi fruit, peeled and sliced
¼ Galia melon, peeled and sliced
200g/7oz fresh lychees, peeled and pitted
2 star fruit, chopped
120g/4¼oz seedless green grapes,
    chopped

1 To make the dressing, put the teabag and 140ml/4½fl oz/generous ½ cup boiling water in a heatproof bowl and leave to infuse for 5 minutes. Remove the tea bag from the water and discard. Leave the water to cool completely, then cover and chill in the fridge for 30 minutes.

2 Stir in the lime juice, agave syrup and mirin and chill for a further 10 minutes. Equally divide the fruit into 4 glasses. Drizzle one-quarter of the dressing over the top of each portion and serve.

Nutritional analysis per serving: Calories 86.2kcal **Protein** 1.3g **Carbohydrates** 21.4g **Fat** 0g

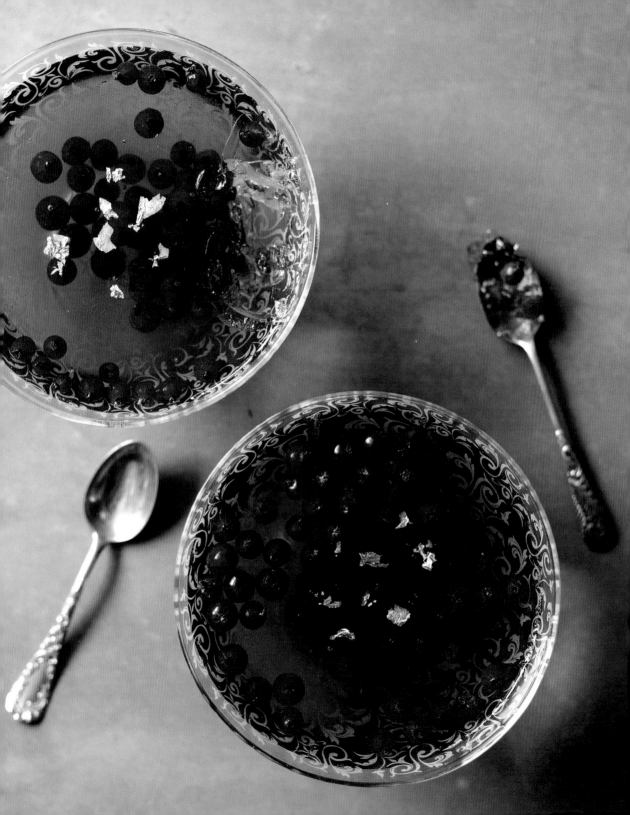

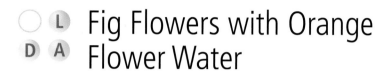

Fig Flowers with Orange Flower Water

MAKES: 4 servings
PREPARATION TIME: 10 minutes

2 tbsp orange flower water
2 tbsp agave syrup
8 figs
2 tbsp roasted salted pistachios,
   shelled and roughly chopped

1 Put the orange flower water and agave syrup in a small bowl and briefly whisk until combined.

2 Using a sharp knife, cut a cross in the top of each fig and pinch the bases so they open out like the petals of a flower. Divide the figs into 4 equal portions. Sprinkle with pistachios, drizzle with the orange flower dressing and serve.

Nutritional analysis per serving: Calories 127kcal **Protein** 3.3g **Carbohydrates** 103.2g **Fat** 0g

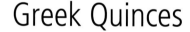
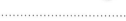

Greek Quinces

MAKES: 4 servings
PREPARATION TIME: 5 minutes, plus 10 minutes soaking
COOKING TIME: 2 hours

1 tbsp raisins
2 tbsp brandy
1 tbsp chopped walnuts
½ tsp ground cinnamon
100ml/3½fl oz/generous ⅓ cup
   agave syrup
20g/¾oz butter, softened
2 quinces or pears
4 tbsp reduced-fat Greek yogurt,
   to serve

1 Preheat the oven to 180°C/350°F/Gas 4. Soak the raisins in the brandy for 10 minutes until softened.

2 Put the walnuts, cinnamon, agave syrup, butter and the raisins and soaking brandy in a bowl and mix until well combined. Core and halve the quinces and arrange, cut-side up, in a baking dish. Spoon one-quarter of the walnut mixture into each quince half, pressing it down into the cavities with the back of a metal spoon.

3 Pour 250ml/9fl oz/1 cup water into the dish, cover with foil and bake for 2 hours until the quinces are soft but retaining their shape. If necessary, occasionally add a little more water to the dish to prevent the quinces from drying out. (Almost all of the water should have evaporated by the end of the cooking time.) Remove from the oven and divide into 4 equal portions, reserving any cooking juices. Top each serving with yogurt, drizzle with cooking juices and serve.

Nutritional analysis per serving: Calories 232kcal **Protein** 2.5g **Carbohydrates** 26.8g **Fat** 6.3g

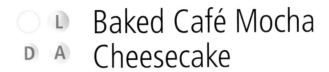

Baked Café Mocha Cheesecake

MAKES: 8 servings
PREPARATION TIME: 15 minutes
COOKING TIME: 35 minutes

Cheesecake seems sinful, but this one is made from cottage cheese – I know, but bear with me! Cottage cheese is full of protein that balances S Factor hormones, and the oatcake base provides a salty contrast to the sweet mocha filling.

140g/5oz oatcakes
2 tbsp chopped walnuts
25g/1oz butter, softened
300g/10½oz/scant 1¼ cups reduced-fat cottage cheese
60g/2¼oz/scant ⅓ cup stevia-based natural sweetener or xylitol
80g/2¾oz/scant ⅓ cup reduced-fat Greek yogurt, plus 4 tbsp extra to serve
4 tsp cornflour
100g/3½oz coffee-flavoured dark chocolate, 70% cocoa solids, broken into squares
2–3 drops of vanilla extract

1 Put the oatcakes in a clean plastic food bag and crush with a rolling pin. Transfer to a bowl, add the walnuts and butter and mix well with a wooden spoon to form a crumbly "dough". Press the dough into a loose-based, 20cm/8in pie dish. Cover and chill in the fridge for 20 minutes.

2 Meanwhile, preheat the oven to 180°C/350°F/Gas 4. Put the cottage cheese, natural sweetener, yogurt and cornflour in a bowl and mix well. Put the chocolate in a heatproof bowl and rest it over a saucepan of gently simmering water, making sure the bottom of the bowl does not touch the water. Heat, stirring occasionally, until the chocolate has melted. Alternatively, melt the chocolate in a glass bowl in the microwave in 10-second spurts – watch carefully to make sure it does not burn. Leave to cool a little.

3 Fold the melted chocolate into the cottage cheese mixture until combined. Spoon the mixture into the pie dish and smooth the surface with the back of a metal spoon. Bake for 20–30 minutes or until the top of the cheesecake has cracked.

4 Mix together the vanilla extract and 4 tablespoons of yogurt in a small bowl. Cut the cheesecake into 8 equal slices, drizzle each slice with the vanilla yogurt and serve hot.

Nutritional analysis per serving: Calories 205kcal **Protein** 15g **Carbohydrates** 13.8g **Fat** 12.5g

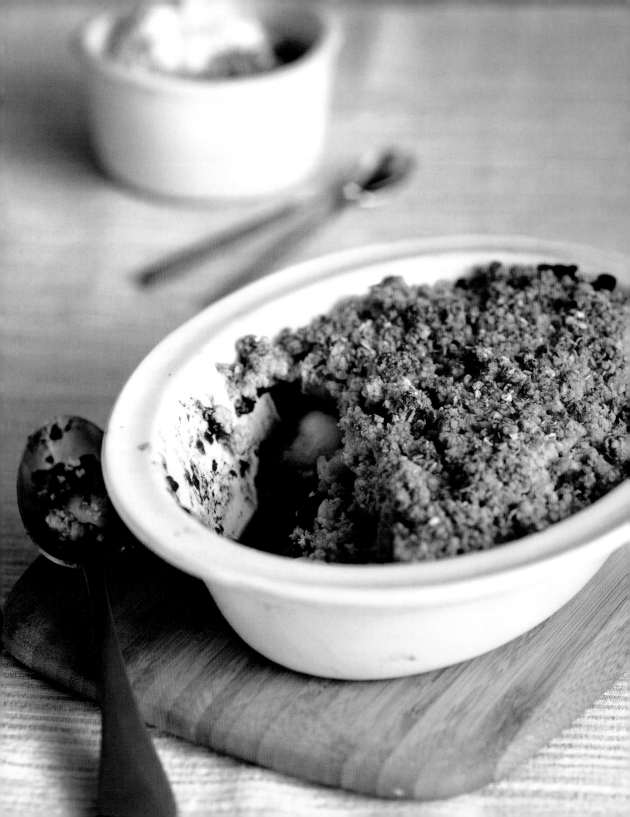

Apple & Blueberry Crumble with Vanilla Tofu Ice Cream

MAKES: 6 servings
PREPARATION TIME: 30 minutes, plus at least 1 hour infusing and at least 1 hour freezing
COOKING TIME: 30 minutes

Let's get the "Tofu! Yuck!" reaction out of the way. Making ice cream from tofu slashes the fat content. You can't taste the tofu and instead you get the delicious flavour of the natural vanilla. This is a sorbet-style ice cream so don't let it freeze too hard.

FOR THE ICE CREAM:
250ml/9fl oz/1 cup skimmed milk or soya milk
100g/3½oz/½ cup stevia-based natural sweetener or xylitol
1 vanilla pod, split lengthways
300g/10½oz silken tofu

FOR THE CRUMBLE:
3 cooking apples
2 tbsp agave syrup
250g/9oz/scant 1⅔ cups fresh blueberries
100g/3½oz/1 cup rolled oats
2 tbsp stevia-based natural sweetener or xylitol
a pinch of ground cinnamon
25g/1oz cold butter, diced

1 To make the ice cream, put the milk, natural sweetener and vanilla pod in a saucepan and heat over a low heat for 3 minutes until the natural sweetener has dissolved. Remove the pan from the heat and leave to stand for at least 1 hour to allow the vanilla flavour to infuse into the milk.

2 Strain the mixture into a blender or food processor, discarding the vanilla pod. Add the tofu and process until smooth. Pour the mixture into an ice cream maker and process according to the manufacturer's instructions. Alternatively, transfer the mixture to a freezer-proof container, cover with a lid and freeze for 1–2 hours until completely frozen.

3 Meanwhile, make the crumble. Preheat the oven to 200°C/400°F/Gas 6. Peel, core and chop the apples. Put the apples and agave syrup in a saucepan and simmer over a medium-low heat for 5 minutes until the apples have softened. Remove the pan from the heat and gently stir in the blueberries. Pour the mixture into a baking dish.

4 Put the oats in a food processor and process until they resemble coarse breadcrumbs. Transfer to a bowl, add the natural sweetener and cinnamon and rub in the butter with your fingertips. Evenly sprinkle the crumble mixture over the top of the fruit and bake for 15–20 minutes until golden. Divide the crumble into 6 equal portions. Serve hot with a scoop of the ice cream.

Nutritional analysis per serving: Calories 184kcal **Protein** 6.2g **Carbohydrates** 24g **Fat** 5.8g

Cherry & Almond Clafoutis

MAKES: 4 servings
PREPARATION TIME: 15 minutes, plus 1 hour steeping
COOKING TIME: 20 minutes

Clafoutis is a French baked custard that's great for all your S Factor hormones. For those wanting to balance dopamine, this recipe is high in protein and the almonds are a great source of tyrosine. Nuts are also beneficial for your adrenals. The natural sugar in the cherries should help to bump up serotonin, too.

150g/5½oz cherries, stoned
1 tsp kirsch
25g/1oz flaked almonds
extra virgin olive oil cooking spray
125ml/4fl oz/½ cup skimmed milk
2 tbsp stevia-based natural sweetener or xylitol
25g/1oz plain wholemeal flour
a pinch of fine sea salt
2 eggs, beaten
2–3 drops of almond extract
4 large pinches of ground cinnamon, for sprinkling

1 Put the cherries and kirsch in a bowl and leave to steep for 1 hour. Meanwhile, heat a non-stick frying pan over a medium-high heat. Dry-fry the almonds for 2 minutes, stirring occasionally, until golden and lightly toasted. Watch carefully so they do not burn. Remove the pan from the heat and leave to cool.

2 Preheat the oven to 200°C/400°F/Gas 6 and mist four 175ml/5½fl oz/⅔-cup ramekins with cooking spray. Put the milk, natural sweetener, flour, salt, eggs and almond extract in a bowl. Using an electric mixer, whisk for 5 minutes, incorporating as much air as possible into the batter, until fluffy and doubled in volume. If using a balloon whisk instead of an electric mixer, whisk for about 12 minutes.

3 Drain the cherries and pour the steeping liquid into the batter. Spoon one-quarter of the cherries into each ramekin and evenly pour the batter over the top. Bake for 10–15 minutes until risen and a skewer inserted into the centre comes out clean. (If the clafoutis start to turn a dark brown colour, cover the ramekins with foil and continue to bake until cooked through). Sprinkle with the toasted almonds and cinnamon and serve warm.

Nutritional analysis per serving: Calories 180kcal **Protein** 5.5g **Carbohydrates** 11g **Fat** 6.2g

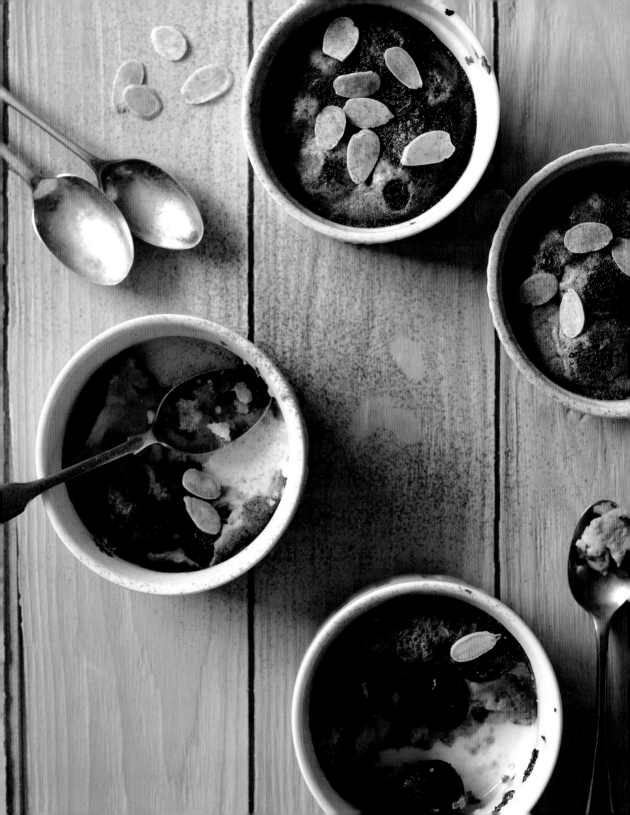

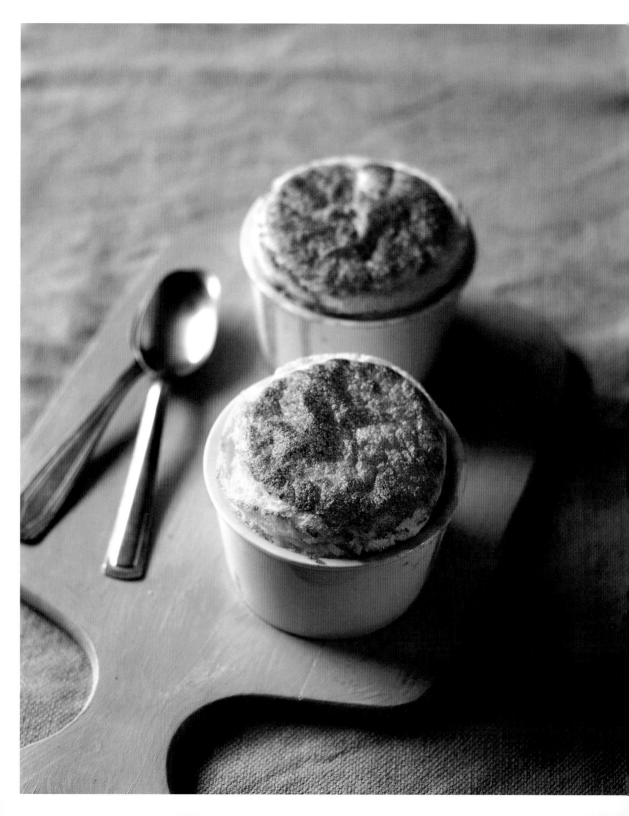

Rhubarb Soufflés

MAKES: 4 servings
PREPARATION TIME: 15 minutes
COOKING TIME: 35 minutes

Rhubarb's slight sharpness, protein-rich eggs and low GI semolina all make these soufflés great for stablizing blood sugar. Normally, this dessert is made with a shedload of sugar, but here I've used natural sweetener so your energy and your S Factor hormones stay balanced.

extra virgin olive oil cooking spray
300g/10½oz pink rhubarb, cut into chunks
3 tbsp stevia-based natural sweetener or xylitol
300ml/10½fl oz/scant 1¼ cups skimmed milk or soya milk
3 tbsp semolina
2 eggs, separated
4 pinches of ground cinnamon

1 Preheat the oven to 180°C/350°F/Gas 4 and mist four 175ml/5½fl oz/⅔-cup ramekins with cooking spray. Put the rhubarb, 2 tablespoons of the natural sweetener and 60ml/2fl oz/¼ cup water in a saucepan. Bring to the boil over a medium-high heat, then reduce the heat to low and simmer, covered, for 5–10 minutes until the rhubarb has softened. Remove the pan from the heat and spoon one-quarter of the mixture into each ramekin. Leave to one side.

2 Pour the milk into another saucepan and heat over a medium-high heat. Bring to just below boiling point, then sprinkle in the semolina and the remaining natural sweetener. Cook, stirring, for 2 minutes until thickened. Remove the pan from the heat, stir in one egg yolk and leave to cool a little. Discard the remaining yolk.

3 Put the egg whites in a clean bowl. Using an electric mixer, whisk until they form stiff peaks, then gently fold them into the semolina mixture, using a metal spoon. Spoon the mixture evenly into the ramekins. Bake for 20 minutes until golden brown and well risen. Remove from the oven, sprinkle each soufflé with a pinch of cinnamon and serve immediately.

Nutritional analysis per serving: Calories 82kcal **Protein** 5.3g **Carbohydrates** 15.8g **Fat** 2.9g

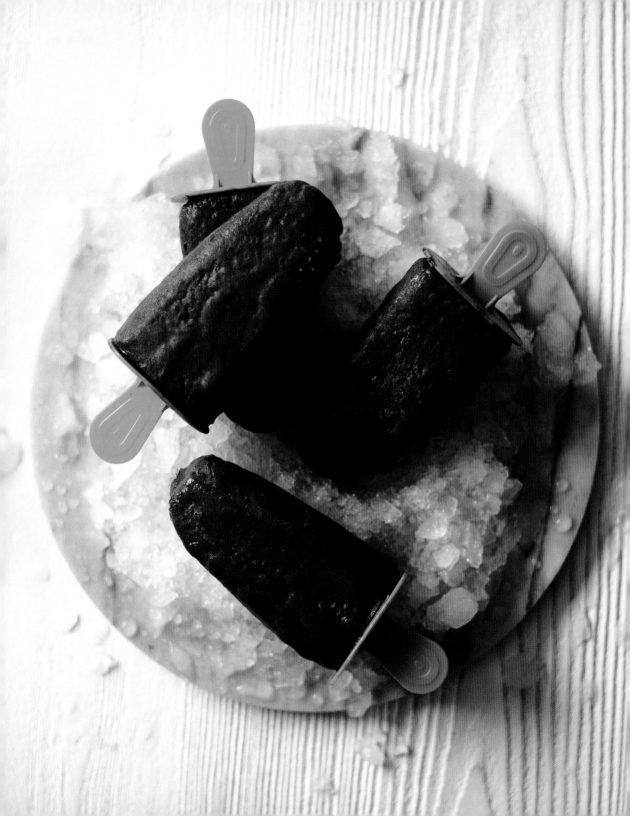

Blackberry Yogurt Lollies

MAKES: 4 servings
PREPARATION TIME: 10 minutes,
plus cooling and at least 2 hours freezing
COOKING TIME: 5 minutes

Most ice cream is a high-fat, high-sugar diet disaster. These lollies have zero fat and are high in protein – the raw material for making diet-tastic S Factor hormones. They're also a gorgeous colour and have a comforting creamy texture, so you'll never know you're eating a diet treat.

80g/2¾oz/generous ⅓ cup stevia-based natural sweetener or xylitol
150g/5½oz/scant 1¼ cups blackberries
120g/4¼oz/scant ½ cup reduced-fat Greek yogurt
juice of 1 lemon

1 Put the natural sweetener and 40ml/1¼fl oz/3 tablespoons water in a saucepan. Heat, stirring, over a low heat until the natural sweetener has dissolved and the mixture is syrupy. Remove the pan from the heat and leave to cool completely.

2 Meanwhile, put the blackberries in a blender or food processor and process to a smooth purée. Using the back of a metal spoon, press the purée through a sieve into a clean bowl. Discard the pulp and pips.

3 Return the blackberry purée to the blender or food processor and add the sweetener syrup, yogurt and lemon juice. Process again until smooth, then pour the mixture into four lolly moulds and freeze for 2–3 hours. When the lollies have completely frozen, remove from the moulds and serve. If the lollies are stuck, briefly hold the moulds under hot running water and carefully remove the lollies.

Nutritional analysis per serving: Calories 23kcal **Protein** 2.6g **Carbohydrates** 2.6g **Fat** 0g

Banana Rice Pudding

MAKES: 6 servings
PREPARATION TIME: 5 minutes
COOKING TIME: 20 minutes

Rice pudding is the ultimate comfort food, but you can basically spread the traditional recipe straight onto your thighs. This one uses high-fibre brown sushi rice and is flavoured with bananas. Bananas are a great source of magnesium – a natural relaxant perfect for getting you ready for bed.

300g/10½oz/scant 1½ cups brown sushi rice
120ml/3¾fl oz/scant ½ cup skimmed milk or soya milk, plus extra if needed
3 tbsp agave syrup
½ tsp ground cinnamon, plus 6 pinches extra for sprinkling
25g/1oz butter
1 large banana, thinly sliced
2 tsp stevia-based natural sweetener or xylitol

1 Put the rice, milk, agave syrup and cinnamon in a saucepan and bring to the boil over a medium-high heat. Reduce the heat to low and simmer for 15–20 minutes until the rice is very soft, adding a little extra milk if the rice looks too dry.

2 Five minutes before serving, melt the butter in a non-stick frying pan over a medium heat. Add the banana and fry for 2 minutes, then sprinkle in the natural sweetener and cook for a further 2 minutes until bubbling. Divide the rice pudding into 6 equal portions. Top with the caramelized banana, sprinkle with cinnamon and serve.

Nutritional analysis per serving: Calories 249kcal **Protein** 4.2g **Carbohydrates** 45g **Fat** 1.8g

Chocolate Yogurt Mousses

MAKES: 4 servings
PREPARATION TIME: 10 minutes,
plus at least 10 minutes chilling
COOKING TIME: 5 minutes

Chocolate mousse usually has that diet-breaking combination of chocolate and cream. The S Factor version uses egg whites and reduced-fat yogurt, so it's protein packed and low in fat. Best of all, it still tastes of yummy chocolate!

150g/5½oz dark chocolate, 70% cocoa solids broken into squares
4 egg whites
1 tbsp stevia-based natural sweetener or xylitol
2 heaped tbsp reduced-fat Greek yogurt
1 tbsp salted pistachios, shelled and chopped, to serve
1 tbsp goji berries, chopped, to serve

1 Put the chocolate in a heatproof bowl and rest it over a saucepan of gently simmering water, making sure the bottom of the bowl does not touch the water. Heat, stirring occasionally, until the chocolate has melted. Alternatively, melt the chocolate in a glass bowl in the microwave in 10-second spurts – watch carefully to make sure it does not burn. Leave to cool a little.

2 Put the egg whites in a clean bowl. Using an electric mixer, whisk until they form stiff peaks. Gently stir in the natural sweetener.

3 Add the yogurt to the melted chocolate and stir until smooth. Using a metal spoon, fold the egg whites into the chocolate mixture, one spoonful at a time, until completely incorporated. Take care not to lose too much volume.

4 Spoon one-quarter of the mousse mixture into each of four glasses or ramekins. Cover with cling film and chill in the fridge for 10–15 minutes until set. Sprinkle each portion with pistachios and goji berries and serve.

Nutritional analysis per serving: Calories 216kcal **Protein** 6.3g **Carbohydrates** 21g **Fat** 11.3g

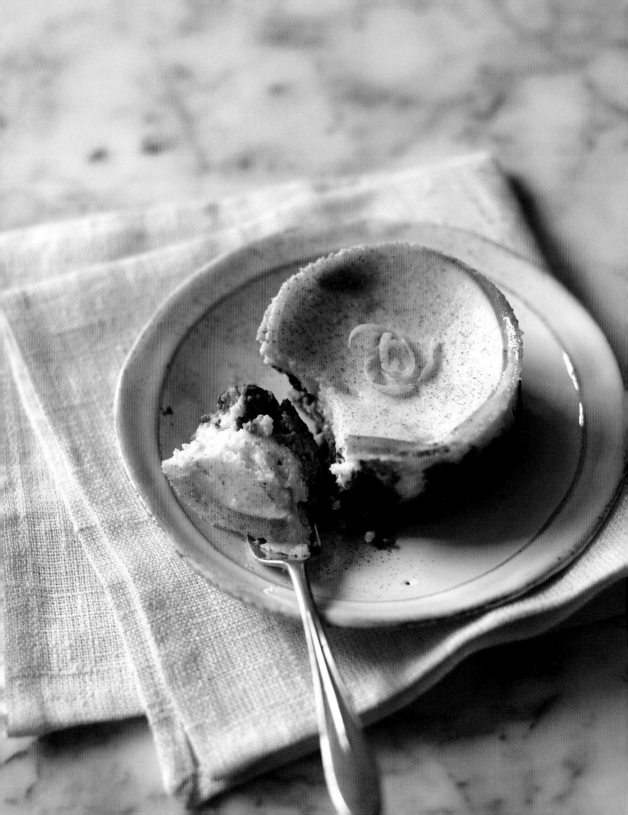

Old-Fashioned Lemon Cheesecakes

MAKES: 4 servings
PREPARATION TIME: 10 minutes, plus 40 minutes chilling
COOKING TIME: 30 minutes

This is a real old-fashioned pud-style snack. It's packed with protein, thanks to the pecans, cottage cheese and yogurt, so it helps to balance blood sugar, which in turn balances all of the S Factor hormones.

extra virgin olive oil cooking spray
12 dates, pitted and chopped
20g/¾oz/scant ¼ cup pecans, chopped
100ml/3½fl oz/generous ⅓ cup skimmed milk or soya milk
1 tsp vanilla extract
300g/10½oz/scant 1¼ cups cottage cheese
60g/2¼oz/scant ⅓ cup stevia-based natural sweetener or xylitol
juice of ½ lemon
80g/2¾oz/scant ⅓ cup reduced-fat Greek yogurt
4 tsp cornflour
1 handful of sultanas
4 pinches of ground cinnamon, to serve
strips of lemon zest, to serve

1 Mist four 6cm/2½in presentation rings with cooking spray. Place the presentation rings on a baking sheet lined with baking parchment. Put the dates, pecans, milk and vanilla extract in a blender or food processor and process until a smooth paste forms. Spoon one-quarter of the paste into each presentation ring. Cover and chill in the fridge for 40 minutes.

2 Preheat the oven to 180°C/350°F/Gas 4. Clean the blender or food processor. Add all of the remaining ingredients, except the sultanas, and process until smooth. Stir in the sultanas, then spoon the mixture evenly into the presentation rings. Level the surface of each cheesecake with the back of a metal spoon, then bake for 30 minutes until golden.

3 Remove from the oven and leave to cool a little. Transfer each presentation ring to a plate, then carefully run a knife around the inside of each presentation ring to loosen the cheesecakes on to the plates. Sprinkle each portion with cinnamon and decorate with strips of lemon zest. Serve warm.

Nutritional analysis per serving: Calories 173kcal **Protein** 4g **Carbohydrates** 20.3g **Fat** 1.3g

Apricot & Oat Cookies

MAKES: 4 servings (8 cookies)
PREPARATION TIME: 15 minutes, plus cooling
COOKING TIME: 10 minutes

Oats are great for balancing leptin because they're high in fibre and resistant starch, both of which help you feel full – a sensation that those with leptin problems struggle to achieve.

2 tsp butter
40g/1½oz/scant ¼ cup stevia-based natural sweetener or xylitol
1 egg, beaten
2–3 drops vanilla extract
40g/1½oz/heaped ¼ cup wholemeal flour
75g/2½oz/¾ cup porridge oats
25g/1oz dried apricots, finely chopped
¼ tsp baking powder
a pinch of ground cinnamon

1 Preheat the oven to 180°C/350°F/ Gas 4 and a line a baking sheet with baking parchment. Put the butter and natural sweetener in a mixing bowl and beat until light and fluffy, then beat in the egg and vanilla extract. Add all of the remaining ingredients and beat slowly with a wooden spoon until just combined. Take care not to overmix.

2 Divide the mixture into 8 equal portions, then shape each one into a ball and place on the baking sheet, spacing them well apart, then flatten each ball slightly. Bake for 10 minutes until golden.

3 Remove from the oven and transfer to a wire rack. Leave to cool completely, then serve.

Nutritional analysis per serving: Calories 152kcal **Protein** 4.8g **Carbohydrates** 23g **Fat** 5.2g

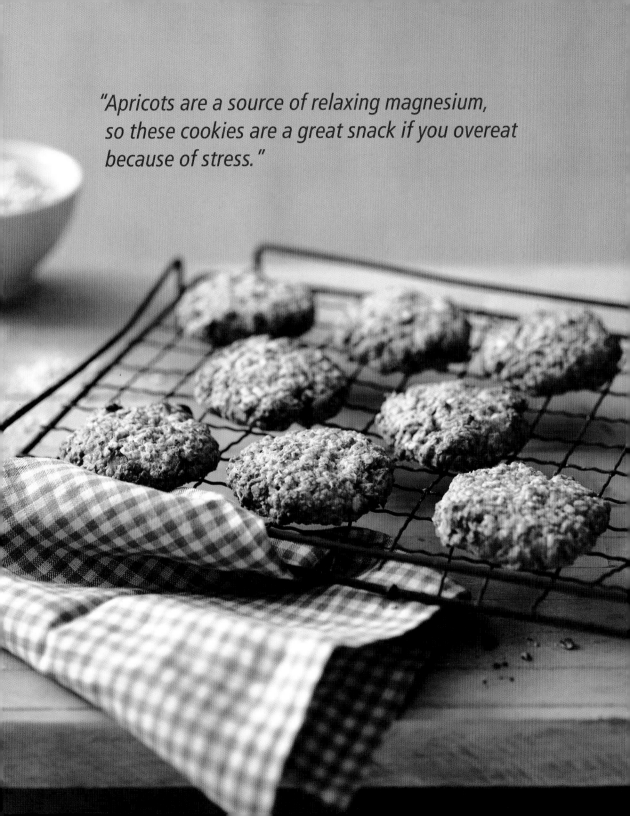

"Apricots are a source of relaxing magnesium, so these cookies are a great snack if you overeat because of stress."

Rainbow Macaroons

MAKES: 12 servings (24 macaroons)
PREPARATION TIME: 1 hour, plus 15 minutes standing
COOKING TIME: 30 minutes

Macaroons are the perfect serotonin-balancing evening snack – the mini-sugar hit stimulates the release of the hormone insulin, which helps serotonin reach the brain and do its job properly. The ground almonds will also help your adrenals.

3 egg whites
a pinch of fine sea salt
75g/2½oz/scant ⅓ cup caster sugar
1 tsp vanilla extract
pink, purple, blue and yellow food colouring
125g/4½oz/1 cup icing sugar
125g/4½oz/1¼ cups ground almonds
120g/4¼oz/scant ½ cup reduced-fat cream cheese
2 tsp stevia-based natural sweetener or xylitol
2–3 drops of vanilla extract

1 Line two baking sheets with baking parchment. Whisk the egg whites and salt in a clean bowl until the egg whites form soft peaks. Add the caster sugar and vanilla extract and whisk until thick and glossy. Divide the egg whites into four clean bowls and mix 1 drop of one food colouring into each bowl to make up pink, purple, blue and yellow mixtures.

2 In another bowl, mix together the icing sugar and ground almonds. Using a spatula, gradually fold one-quarter of the ground almond mixture into each bowl of egg whites, folding until the macaroon mixtures are shiny and stiff.

3 Preheat the oven to 140°C/275°F/Gas 1. Spoon one of the mixtures into a piping bag with a plain nozzle. Twisting the bag as necessary, neatly pipe 12, 4cm/1½in circles onto one of the baking sheets, spacing the circles well apart. Using the back of a metal spoon, flatten the top of each circle. Repeat with the remaining macaroon mixtures until you have 48 circles, cleaning the piping bag before piping each batch. Leave to stand at room temperature for 10–15 minutes until the tops of the macaroons are dry to the touch, then bake for 30 minutes until crisp. Remove from the oven and leave to cool completely.

4 Meanwhile, make the filling. In a mixing bowl, beat together the cream cheese, natural sweetener and vanilla extract. Divide the mixture into four clean bowls and mix 1 drop of one of the food colouring into each bowl to make up pink, purple, blue and yellow fillings.

5 When the macaroons have cooled completely, spread a little filling onto one macaroon, then sandwich together with another macaroon. Repeat with the remaining macaroons, dividing the fillings evenly between them, then serve.

Nutritional analysis per serving: Calories 158kcal **Protein** 4g **Carbohydrates** 89g **Fat** 2g

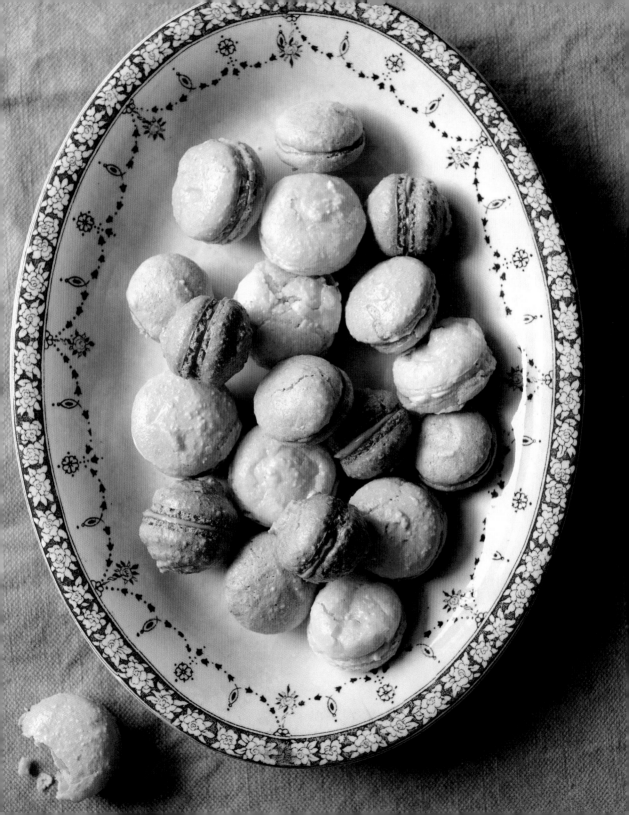

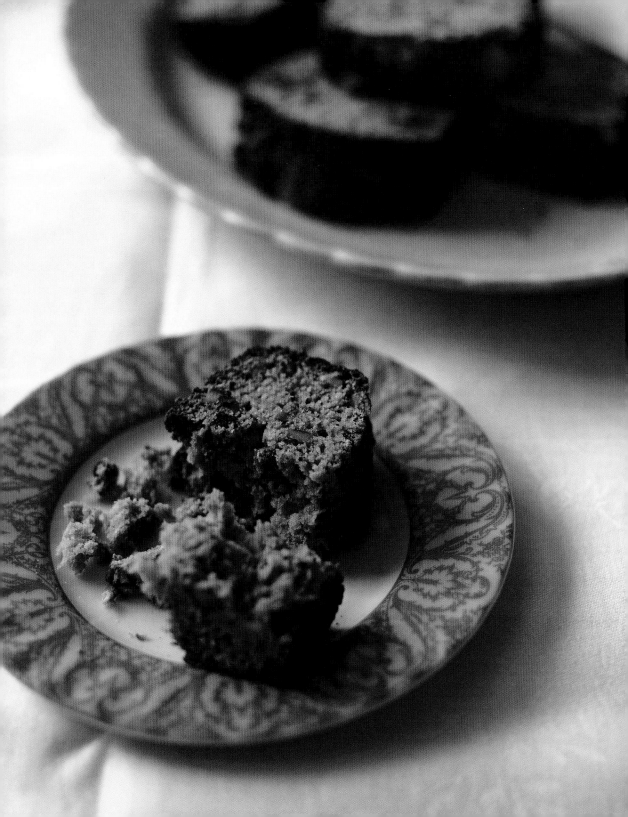

S L D A Banana, Apple & Walnut Bread

MAKES: 6 servings
PREPARATION TIME: 20 minutes. plus cooling
COOKING TIME: 35 minutes

Bananas have had such bad press for being sugary, but unripe ones are a powerhouse of leptin-friendly resistant starch. The walnuts will help to balance your dopamine and serotonin, and they'll even nourish your adrenals. And all this in a baked treat!

extra virgin olive oil cooking spray
25g/1oz butter
1 dessert apple, such as Granny Smith or Golden Delicious, peeled, cored and finely chopped
6 tbsp stevia-based natural sweetener or xylitol
50g/1¾oz/heaped ⅓ cup plain white flour
50g/1¾oz/⅓ cup plain wholemeal flour
1¼ tsp baking powder
¼ tsp bicarbonate of soda
a pinch ground cinnamon
1 egg white
1 large unripe banana, finely chopped
2 tbsp chopped walnuts

1 Preheat the oven to 180°C/350°F/Gas 4 and mist a 450g/1lb loaf tin with cooking spray, then line with baking parchment.

2 Melt the butter in a non-stick frying pan over a medium-low heat. Add the apple and cook for 2 minutes, then sprinkle in 1 teaspoon of natural sweetener and cook for a further 1 minute until the natural sweetener has dissolved. Remove from the heat and leave to cool a little, then mash with a fork or purée with a hand blender until smooth.

3 Sift the flours, baking powder, bicarbonate of soda and cinnamon into a large mixing bowl. Add the remaining natural sweetener, apple purée and all of the remaining ingredients and beat slowly with a wooden spoon until just combined. Take care not to overmix. Pour the mixture into the loaf tin and level the surface, using a clean knife.

4 Bake for 30 minutes until a skewer inserted in the centre comes out clean. Remove from the oven and leave to cool in the tin for 5 minutes, then transfer to a wire rack and leave to cool completely. Slice into 6 slices and serve.

Nutritional analysis per serving: Calories 112kcal **Protein** 2.8g **Carbohydrates** 16.7g **Fat** 4.2g

Chilli Pitta Crisps

MAKES: 6 servings
PREPARATION TIME: 5 minutes
COOKING TIME: 15 minutes

4 wholemeal pitta breads, split
   lengthways and cut into small
   triangles
extra virgin olive oil cooking spray
4 tsp mild chilli powder

1 Preheat the oven to 180°C/350°F/Gas 4. Spread the triangles of pitta in a single layer over a baking tray and mist with cooking spray.

2 Dust with 2 teaspoons of the chilli powder. Cook for 5–10 minutes, then turn over, mist again with cooking spray and dust with the remaining chilli powder. Cook for a further 5 minutes until crisp. Remove from the oven and leave to cool a little. Divide into 6 equal portions and serve warm.

Nutritional analysis per serving: Calories 170kcal **Protein** 6g **Carbohydrates** 36.6g **Fat** 9.3g

Indian-Style Trail Mix

MAKES: 10 servings
PREPARATION TIME: 10 minutes
COOKING TIME: 45 minutes

1–2 tbsp extra virgin olive oil
1 tbsp agave syrup
1 tsp Worcestershire sauce
a pinch of fine sea salt
1 tbsp mild curry powder
2 wholemeal pitta breads, cut into
   matchsticks
100g/3½oz/heaped 3 cups
   unsweetened puffed brown rice
150g/5½oz salted pretzels, chopped
60g/2¼oz chopped dried mango

1 Preheat the oven to 200°C/400°F/Gas 6 and line a baking tin with baking parchment. Heat the oil in a non-stick frying pan over a medium heat. Add the agave syrup, Worcestershire sauce, salt and curry powder and cook, stirring, for 10 seconds. Remove the pan from heat. Gradually add the pitta bread sticks, puffed brown rice and pretzels to the mixture and toss until well coated.

2 Pour the mixture into the baking tin, turn the oven down to 100°C/200°F/Gas ½ and cook for 40 minutes until golden. Remove from the oven and transfer to a large bowl. Stir in the mango and leave to cool completely. Divide into 10 equal portions and serve at room temperature.

Nutritional analysis per serving: Calories 181kcal **Protein** 4.3g **Carbohydrates** 33g **Fat** 2.8g

Tangy Toasted Seeds

MAKES: 6 servings
PREPARATION TIME: 5 minutes
COOKING TIME: 45 minutes

4 tbsp soy sauce
1 tsp ground ginger
4 tsp agave syrup
80g/2¾oz/scant ½ cup pumpkin seeds
80g/2¾oz/scant ⅔ cup sunflower seeds

1 Preheat the oven to 180°C/350°F/Gas 4 and line a baking tray with baking parchment. Mix together the soy sauce, ginger and agave syrup in a small bowl. Put the seeds in a bowl, pour over the soy dressing and toss well, making sure the seeds are well coated.

2 Spread the seeds in an even layer over the baking tray. Cook for 45 minutes, stirring occasionally, until crisp and toasted. Remove from the oven and leave to cool a little. Divide into 6 equal portions and serve.

Nutritional analysis per serving: Calories 184kcal **Protein** 5.2g **Carbohydrates** 12.6g **Fat** 12.6g

Spiced Pecans

MAKES: 12 servings
PREPARATION TIME: 5 minutes
COOKING TIME: 30 minutes

1 tbsp extra virgin rapeseed oil
1 tbsp chilli powder
1 tsp fine sea salt
400g/14oz pecan halves

1 Preheat the oven to 180°C/350°F/Gas 4 and line a baking tray with baking parchment. Mix together the oil, chilli powder and salt in a bowl. Add the pecans and toss well, making sure the pecans are well coated.

2 Spread the pecans in a single layer over the baking tray. Cook for 20–30 minutes, turning once, until crisp. Remove from the oven and leave to cool completely. Divide into 12 equal portions and serve.

Nutritional analysis per serving: Calories 250kcal **Protein** 3g **Carbohydrates** 1.9g **Fat** 27g

Spiced Hot Chocolate

MAKES: 4 servings
PREPARATION TIME: 10 minutes,
plus 10 minutes infusing
COOKING TIME: 15 minutes

1 red chilli, scored with stalk intact
2 tsp stevia-based natural sweetener
  or xylitol
750ml/26fl oz/3 cups skimmed milk or
  soya milk
100g/3½oz dark chocolate, 70%
  cocoa solids, broken into squares
a pinch of ground ginger
a pinch of ground cinnamon
4 pinches of ground paprika

1   Put the chilli, natural sweetener and milk in a saucepan and bring to a simmer, stirring occasionally, over a medium-low heat. Remove the pan from the heat and leave to stand for 10 minutes to allow the chilli flavour to infuse into the milk.

2   Meanwhile, put the chocolate in a heatproof bowl and rest it over a saucepan of gently simmering water, making sure the bottom of the bowl does not touch the water. Heat, stirring occasionally, until the chocolate has melted. Alternatively, melt the chocolate in a glass bowl in the microwave in 10-second spurts – watch carefully to make sure it does not burn.

3   Remove the chilli from the milk and discard. Add the melted chocolate, ginger and cinnamon to the milk mixture. Simmer, stirring, over a medium-low heat until the chocolate has completely dissolved and the mixture is smooth. Divide into four cups, sprinkle each serving with a pinch of paprika and serve hot.

Nutritional analysis per serving: Calories 185kcal **Protein** 7.8g **Carbohydrates** 20.5g
Fat 8.3g

Barley Bedtime Drink

MAKES: 4 servings
PREPARATION TIME: 10 minutes
COOKING TIME: 35 minutes

250g/9oz/scant 1¼ cups pearl barley
750ml/26fl oz/3 cups semi-skimmed
  milk or soya milk
6 cardamom pods, crushed
a pinch of freshly grated nutmeg
zest of ½ orange, reserving 1 tsp
2 tbsp agave syrup

1   Put the pearl barley, milk, cardamom pods and nutmeg in a saucepan and stir in the orange zest. Bring to the boil over a medium-low heat, then reduce the heat to low and simmer for 30 minutes until thickened.

2   Strain through a sieve into a clean bowl, discarding the solids. Add the agave syrup and stir until dissolved. Divide into four cups, sprinkle with the reserved orange zest and serve hot.

Nutritional analysis per serving: Calories 132kcal **Protein** 8.3g **Carbohydrates** 10.2g
Fat 5g

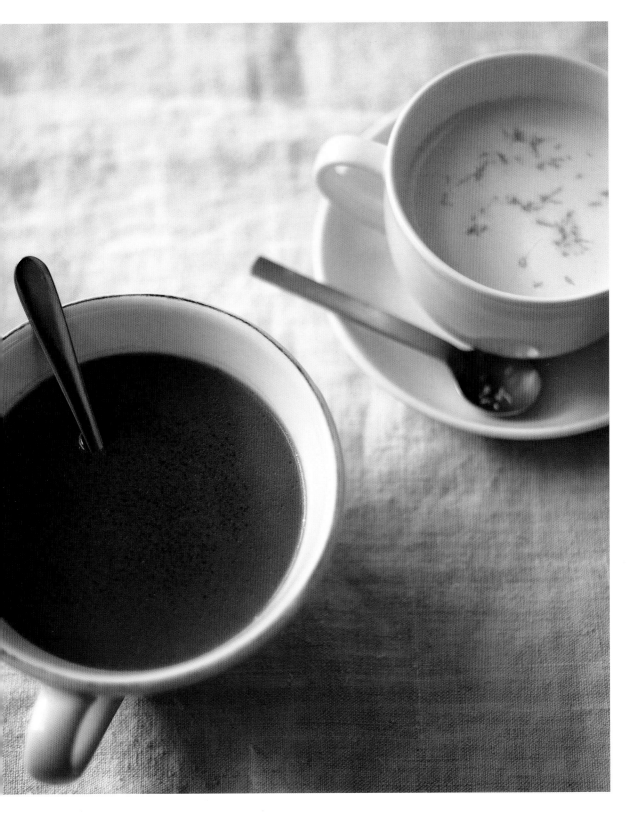

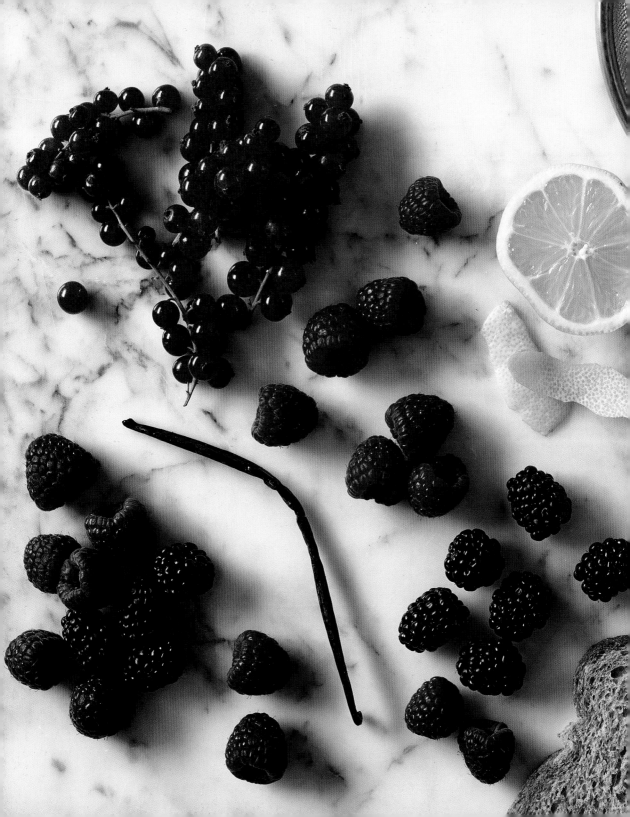

The S Factor Lifetime Diet

You've reached your goal weight. Now what? Most diets scramble your S Factor hormones and send you straight back to your old eating habits. The S Factor diet has balanced your S Factor hormones, so you won't have that end-of-diet, "I HAVE TO EAT A CAKE NOW", feeling.

To help you maintain your weight loss, the S Factor Lifetime Diet follows the same hormone-friendly principles and gives you new ideas (and a few more calories) to play with. Follow one of the 2-day sample meal plans or construct your own menu by selecting recipes from chapters 2 and 3 with your hormone symbol. Always stick to around 1500–2500 calories per day. Keep up the good work and enjoy!

Lifetime Diet Meal Plans

Serotonin

DAY 1

Breakfast Coconut French Toast with Warm Berry "Compôte" (see page 129)

Lunch Brown Rice Sushi (see page 136)

Dinner Japanese Tuna Parcels with Wilted Greens (see page 143), Mini Mango & Passion Fruit Pavlovas (see page 144)

S Factor Snack Chocolate-Dipped Pretzels (see page 156)

DAY 2

Breakfast Waffles with Strawberries & Bananas (see page 126)

Lunch Latkes with Smoked Mackerel & Dill Crème Fraîche (see page 134)

Dinner Chicken Tikka Masala (see page 139), Baby Summer Puddings (see page 147)

S Factor Snack High-Protein Cranberry Brownies (see page 154)

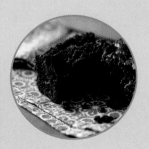

Leptin

DAY 1

Breakfast Waffles with Strawberries & Bananas (see page 126)

Lunch Brown Rice Sushi (see page 136)

Dinner Fish, Chips & Mushy Peas (see page 142), American-Style Pumpkin Pie (see page 149)

S Factor Snack Sweet Potato & Pecan Cupcakes (see page 153)

DAY 2

Breakfast Coconut French Toast with Warm Berry "Compôte" (see page 129)

Lunch Super Scandi (see page 135)

Dinner Chicken Tikka Masala (see page 139), Mini Mango & Passion Fruit Pavlovas (see page 144)

S Factor Snack Chocolate-Dipped Pretzels (see page 156)

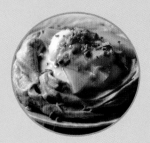

Dopamine

DAY 1

Breakfast Persian Baked Eggs (see page 130)

Lunch Latkes with Smoked Mackerel & Dill Crème Fraîche (see page 134)

Dinner Herb-Crusted Pork with Roast Potatoes (see page 140), American-Style Pumpkin Pie (see page 149)

S Factor Snack High-Protein Cranberry Brownies (see page 154)

DAY 2

Breakfast Waffles with Strawberries & Bananas (see page 126)

Lunch Turkey Burgers (see page 133)

Dinner Chicken Tikka Masala (see page 139), Mini Mango & Passion Fruit Pavlovas (see page 144)

S Factor Snack Almond Butter Cookies (see page 157)

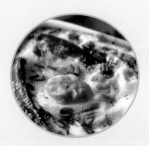

Adrenals

DAY 1

Breakfast Persian Baked Eggs (see page 130)

Lunch Latkes with Smoked Mackerel & Dill Crème Fraîche (see page 134)

Dinner Herb-Crusted Pork with Roast Potatoes (see page 140), Chocolate & Avocado Truffles (see page 150)

S Factor Snack Almond Butter Cookies (see page 157)

DAY 2

Breakfast Waffles with Strawberries & Bananas (see page 126)

Lunch Super Scandi (see page 135)

Dinner Fish, Chips & Mushy Peas (see page 142), Mini Mango & Passion Fruit Pavlovas (see page 144)

S Factor Snack Sweet Potato & Pecan Cupcakes (see page 153)

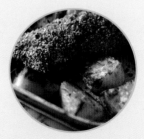

⒮ ⓛ Waffles with Strawberries
⒟ ⓐ & Bananas

MAKES: 4 servings
PREPARATION TIME: 15 minutes
COOKING TIME: 15 minutes

Waffles don't sound like diet food, but if you swap white flour for a mix of soy and wholemeal flours and replace the sugar with natural sweetener, you've actually got a healthy breakfast.

50g/1¾oz/⅓ cup wholemeal self-raising flour
50g/1¾oz/heaped ⅓ cup soya flour
1 tsp baking powder
½ tsp salt
60g/2¼oz/scant ⅓ cup stevia-based natural sweetener or xylitol
2 eggs, lightly beaten
175g/6oz/scant ¾ cup quark or reduced-fat fromage frais
90ml/3fl oz/⅓ cup + 1 tbsp skimmed milk or soy milk
extra virgin olive oil cooking spray
2 bananas, sliced, to serve
175g/6oz strawberries, hulled and halved, to serve
3 tbsp reduced-fat Greek yogurt, to serve
1 tsp agave syrup, to serve
cinnamon, to serve (optional)

1 Preheat the oven to 100°C/200°F/Gas ½. Sift the flours, baking powder and salt into a large mixing bowl. Mix the natural sweetener into the flour mixture. In another bowl, whisk the eggs until frothy, then add the quark and milk and stir until combined.

2 Make a well in the centre of the flour mixture and add the egg mixture. Beat slowly with a wooden spoon to draw in the flours to make a thick, smooth batter.

3 Mist a waffle maker with cooking spray and preheat to medium. Alternatively, mist a waffle iron with cooking spray and heat over a medium heat. Pour one-quarter of the batter into the waffle iron to make a waffle, but take care not to overfill the mould. Cook for about 3–4 minutes until golden and cooked through. Transfer to a wire rack and keep warm in the oven while you repeat with the remaining batter to make 4 waffles, misting the waffle maker or iron with cooking spray before cooking each waffle. Top each waffle with one-quarter of the bananas, strawberries, yogurt and agave syrup. Sprinkle with cinnamon, if you like, and serve.

Nutritional analysis per serving: Calories 230kcal **Protein** 11.4g **Carbohydrates** 21.4g **Fat** 6g

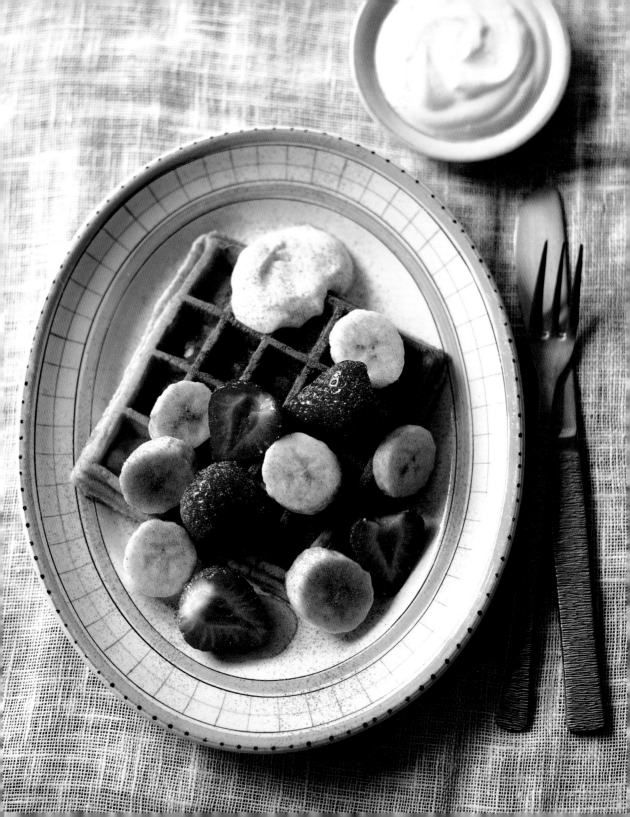

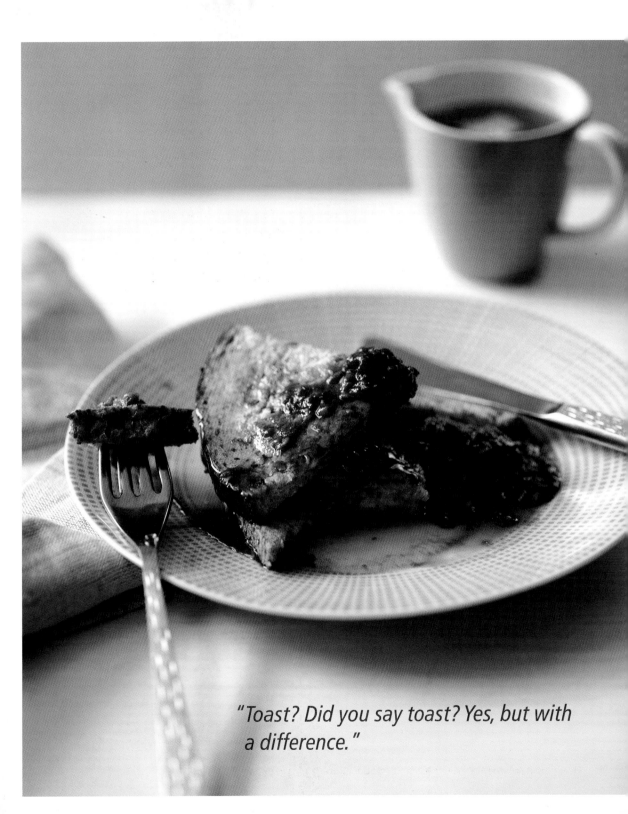

"Toast? Did you say toast? Yes, but with a difference."

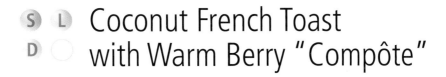

Coconut French Toast with Warm Berry "Compôte"

MAKES: 4 servings
PREPARATION TIME: 10 minutes
COOKING TIME: 15 minutes

The S Factor diet doesn't stop you enjoying toast, but you'll be adding some protein by dipping the bread in egg. Not only will this breakfast help to balance your blood sugar and S Factor hormones, it will also reduce those mid-morning sugar cravings that derail so many diets.

200g/7oz raspberries, blackberries, redcurrants or other berries
2 eggs, beaten
60ml/2fl oz/¼ cup skimmed milk or soya milk
4 thin slices of oatmeal bread or wholemeal bread
50g/1¾oz desiccated coconut
extra virgin olive oil cooking spray
4 tbsp agave syrup

1 Preheat the oven to 100°C/200°F/Gas ½. Put the raspberries in a saucepan and cook over a medium-low heat for 5 minutes until softened. Remove from the heat and mash coarsely with the back of a wooden spoon. Cover with a lid and keep warm.

2 Put the eggs and milk in a large, shallow bowl and beat well. Dip the slices of bread into the mixture until completely coated, then evenly sprinkle the coconut over each slice.

3 Mist a large, non-stick frying pan with cooking spray and heat over a medium heat until smoking. Working in batches, cook the bread for 2 minutes on each side until golden. Keep warm in the oven while you repeat with the remaining dipped bread, misting the pan again with cooking spray before cooking each batch. Spoon one-quarter of the raspberry "compôte" over the top of each serving, drizzle with agave syrup and serve hot.

Nutritional analysis per serving: Calories 490kcal **Protein** 8.1g **Carbohydrates** 29g **Fat** 11.6g

Persian Baked Eggs

MAKES: 4 servings
PREPARATION TIME: 15 minutes
COOKING TIME: 40 minutes

This might not seem like a breakfast dish, but similar recipes are eaten in the morning all over the Middle East. It does require a bit of preparation and time in the oven, so it works best at the weekend when you're not dashing out the door. It delivers a big hit of protein for a dish with very few carbs, so this is best for Dopaminers.

extra virgin olive oil cooking spray
1 red pepper, deseeded and finely sliced
1 green pepper, deseeded and finely sliced
2 garlic cloves, chopped
1 red chilli, deseeded and chopped
400g/14oz/scant 1²/₃ cups tinned chopped tomatoes
1 tsp caraway seeds
1 tsp harissa
a pinch of paprika
a pinch of ground cumin
4 eggs
1 tbsp chopped chives
4 thin slices of rye bread, toasted, to serve

1 Preheat the oven to 180°C/350°F/Gas 4 and mist a non-stick frying pan with cooking spray. Cook the peppers over a medium heat for 10 minutes until softened. Stir in the garlic and chilli and cook for a further 2 minutes. Add the chopped tomatoes, caraway seeds, harissa and spices. Reduce the heat to low and simmer for 10 minutes until thickened.

2 Pour one-quarter of the tomato mixture into each of four 9 x 9cm/3½ x 3½in square ramekins. With the back of a spoon, make a deep hole in the centre of each dish and crack an egg into each hole. Bake for 15 minutes until the egg whites are cooked through. Sprinkle with chives and serve each portion with one slice of rye toast.

Nutritional analysis per serving: Calories 184kcal **Protein** 7g **Carbohydrates** 9g **Fat** 5.5g

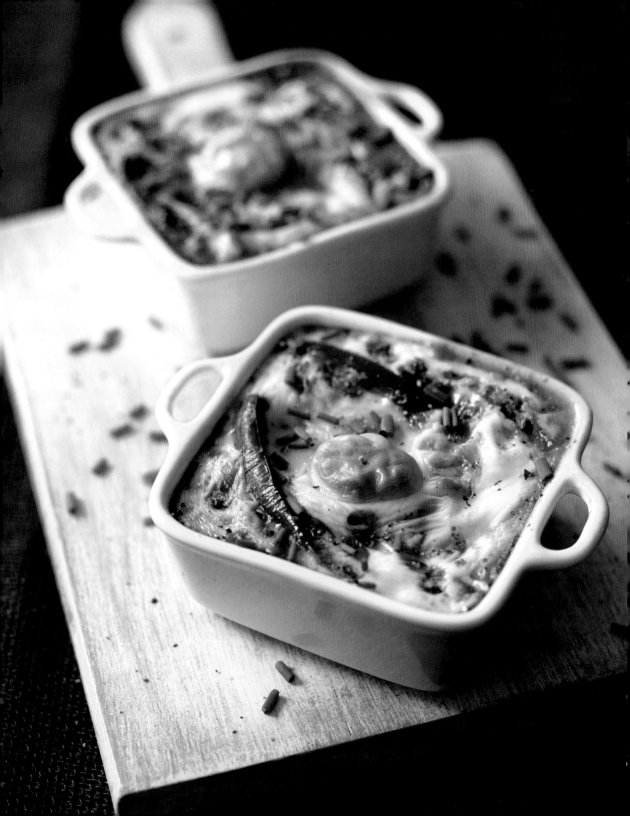

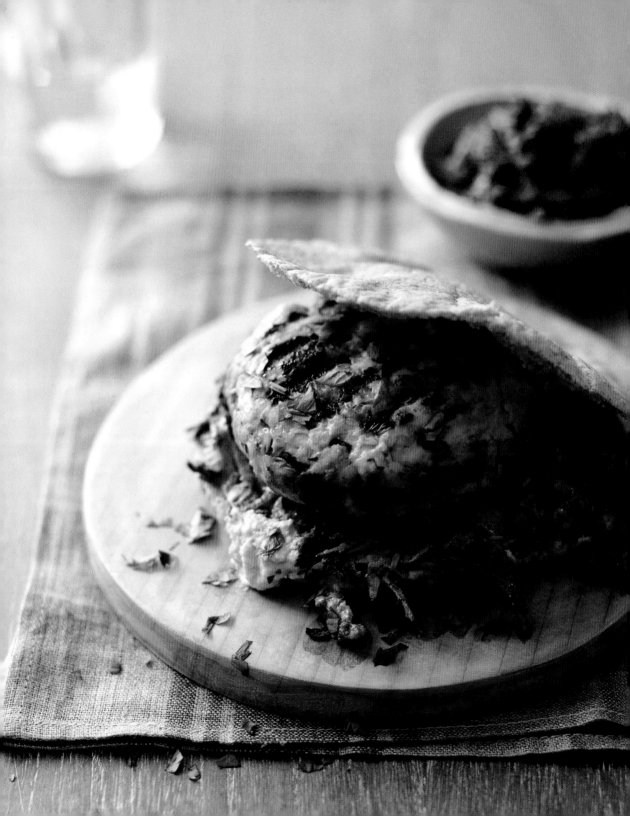

Turkey Burgers

MAKES: 4 servings
PREPARATION TIME: 40 minutes, plus 20 chilling
COOKING TIME: 10 minutes

Bread can be a huge pitfall (you eat a slice and it's so delicious you just keep going), but pitta breads are much easier to portion control. With the protein-rich turkey and the healthy fats from the walnuts, this is a really healthy balanced meal.

440g/15½oz turkey breast, cut into chunks or turkey mince
4 spring onions, chopped
2 tbsp sesame seeds
a splash of soy sauce
1 handful of chopped coriander leaves, plus 1 tbsp extra to serve
1 apple
extra virgin olive oil cooking spray
fine sea salt and freshly ground black pepper
4 wholemeal pitta breads, split, to serve

FOR THE MAYONNAISE:
300g/10½oz silken tofu, roughly chopped
1 garlic clove, peeled
1 large handful of chopped basil leaves
1 tbsp Dijon mustard
1 tbsp red wine vinegar
a pinch of stevia-based natural sweetener or xylitol

FOR THE COLESLAW:
2 carrots, grated
25g/1oz chopped walnuts
¼ red cabbage, grated
3 tbsp reduced-fat Greek yogurt
juice of ½ lemon

1 Put the turkey in a food processor and process until roughly chopped. Transfer to a mixing bowl and add the spring onions, sesame seeds, soy sauce and coriander. Season with salt and pepper and mix until well combined. Using your hands, divide the mixture into 4 equal pieces and roll each one into a ball. Press your finger into the centre of each burger ball to make a hollow.

2 Peel, core and grate the apple, then stuff one-quarter of the gratings into each hollow. Fold the turkey mixture around each hollow to cover the apple. Flatten the balls and shape each one into a burger. Cover and chill in the fridge for 20 minutes.

3 Meanwhile, make the mayonnaise and coleslaw. To make the mayonnaise, clean the food processor, then add all of the ingredients and process until smooth. Cover and chill in the fridge until needed. To make the coleslaw, put the carrots, walnuts and cabbage in a bowl. Add the yogurt and lemon juice, season with salt and pepper and mix until well combined. Cover and chill in the fridge until needed.

4 Heat a large griddle pan over a medium-high heat and mist both sides of the burgers with cooking spray. Cook the burgers for 5 minutes on each side until golden and completely cooked through, working in batches if necessary. Split the pitta breads in half and fill each one with 1 burger, 2 tablespoons of coleslaw, 1 tablespoon of mayonnaise and a sprinkle of coriander. Serve warm.

Nutritional analysis per serving: Calories 620.1kcal **Protein** 46g **Carbohydrates** 61.5g **Fat** 16.7g

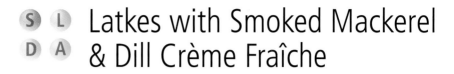

Latkes with Smoked Mackerel & Dill Crème Fraîche

MAKES: 4 servings
PREPARATION TIME: 20 minutes, plus 20 minutes chilling
COOKING TIME: 45 minutes

200g/7oz potatoes, cut into chunks
1 egg, separated
50g/1¾oz/⅓ cup wholemeal flour
a pinch of baking powder
extra virgin olive oil cooking spray
2 smoked mackerel fillets, each about 50g/1¾oz
1 cucumber, grated and chilled, to serve
fine sea salt and freshly ground black pepper

FOR THE CRÈME FRAÎCHE:

150g/5½oz/¾ cup stevia-based natural sweetener or xylitol
150ml/5fl oz/scant ⅔ cup rice vinegar
zest and juice of 2 lemons
200g/7oz/heaped ¾ cup reduced-fat crème fraîche
2 tbsp chopped dill

1   Put the potatoes in a large saucepan and cover with water. Bring to the boil over a medium-high heat, then reduce the heat to low and simmer for 20 minutes until soft. Drain well and transfer to a large bowl. Season with salt and pepper and mash until smooth. Leave to cool completely.

2   Meanwhile, make the crème fraîche. Put the natural sweetener, rice vinegar, lemon zest and juice in a saucepan. Heat over a low heat, stirring, until the natural sweetener has dissolved and the mixture is syrupy. Remove from the heat, transfer to a bowl and leave to cool a little. Stir in the crème fraîche and dill, then cover and chill in the fridge.

3   Preheat the oven to 100°C/200°F/Gas ½. Add the egg yolk, flour and baking powder to the mashed potato. Whisk the egg white in a clean bowl until it forms soft peaks. Using a metal spoon, fold the egg white into the potato mixture until just combined. Using your hands, divide the mixture into 8 equal pieces and shape each one into a flat round. Cover and chill in the fridge for 20 minutes.

4   Mist a large, non-stick frying pan with cooking spray and heat over a medium-high heat. Working in batches, add the latkes to the pan and flatten with a spatula. Cook for 3–5 minutes on each side until golden brown and crisp. Remove from the pan and keep warm in the oven while you repeat with the remaining latkes, misting the pan again with cooking spray before cooking each batch.

5   Meanwhile, wrap the mackerel in foil and transfer to a steamer, or to a colander over a pan with about 5cm/2in water and bring to the boil. Cover and steam for 8–10 minutes until the fish is heated through. Divide the mackerel, latkes and cucumber into 4 equal portions. Top each serving with 1 tablespoon of dill crème fraîche and serve.

Nutritional analysis per serving: Calories 422.5kcal **Protein** 64.3g **Carbohydrates** 23.5g **Fat** 18.3g

Super Scandi

Crispbreads have a lower GI than normal breads and are also higher in resistant starch, so they'll help you feel full and keep your mood and appetite stable for longer. The prep time for the salmon is a bit heart-stopping, but it's worth the wait.

MAKES: 4 servings
PREPARATION TIME: 5 minutes, plus 3 days curing

140g/5oz/scant ¾ cup stevia-based natural sweetener or xylitol
100g/3½oz rock salt
30g/1oz fresh horseradish, peeled and grated
150g/5½oz beetroot, peeled and grated
4 handfuls of chopped dill, plus 1 tsp extra to serve
800g/1lb 12oz skin-on salmon fillet
16 pieces of crispbread, to serve
1 cooked beetroot, diced, to serve

FOR THE TOPPING:
60g/2¼oz/¼ cup reduced-fat crème fraîche
15g/½oz fresh horseradish, peeled and grated
a squeeze of lemon juice

1 Cut two large rectangles of cling film, each large enough to enclose the salmon fillet, and lay the sheets in a double layer over a chopping board. Put the natural sweetener, salt, horseradish, beetroot and dill in a bowl and mix well.

2 Spread half of the dill mixture in an even layer over the cling film. Place the salmon on the cling film, skin-side down, and spread the remaining dill mixture over the top. Wrap the salmon tightly in the cling film, then transfer the parcel to a large container or baking dish. Put a chopping board or tray on top of the salmon and weight it down with bags of dried beans or tins of food. Leave to cure in the fridge for 3 days. Open the parcel every 24 hours and pour off any liquid before rewrapping, turning and weighting down the salmon again.

3 After 3 days, scrape the cure off the salmon and discard. Rinse the salmon under cold running water and pat dry with kitchen paper and transfer to a chopping board. Using a sharp knife, cut the salmon into very thin slices, discarding the skin.

4 To make the topping, mix the crème fraîche, horseradish and lemon juice in a bowl. Divide the crispbreads and salmon into 4 equal portions. Top each crispbread with salmon, followed by 1 tablespoon of the topping and one-quarter of the diced beetroot. Sprinkle with dill and serve.

Nutritional analysis per serving: Calories 369kcal **Protein** 55.1g **Carbohydrates** 16.9g **Fat** 9.4g

Brown Rice Sushi

MAKES: 4 servings
PREPARATION TIME: 20 minutes, plus 30 minutes soaking and 10 minutes chilling
COOKING TIME: 45 minutes

250g/9oz/scant 1½ cups brown sushi rice
80ml/2½fl oz/⅓ cup rice vinegar
2 tbsp stevia-based natural sweetener or xylitol
4 sheets of nori seaweed
1 red pepper, deseeded and cut into matchsticks
1 avocado, peeled, pitted and cut into long slices
fine sea salt and freshly ground black pepper
soy sauce, to serve (optional)
Japanese horseradish, to serve (optional)

FOR THE MAYONNAISE:
190g/6¾oz silken tofu, roughly chopped
1 handful of chopped basil leaves
2 garlic cloves, peeled
1 tbsp extra virgin olive oil
1 tsp wasabi paste, plus extra to serve

1 Rinse the rice under cold running water for 1 minute, then drain and transfer to a heavy-based saucepan. Pour in 535ml/18¾fl oz/scant 2¼ cups cold water and leave to soak for 30 minutes.

2 Meanwhile, make the mayonnaise. Put all of the ingredients, except the wasabi, in a blender or food processor and process until smooth. Transfer to a bowl, season with salt and pepper and stir in the wasabi paste. Cover and chill in the fridge until needed.

3 Bring the soaked rice to the boil over a medium-high heat. Reduce the heat to low, cover with a tight-fitting lid and simmer for 40 minutes until all the water has been absorbed. Remove the pan from the heat and leave to stand, covered, for 10 minutes. Put the vinegar and natural sweetener in a saucepan and heat over a medium heat. Cook, stirring, until the natural sweetener dissolves. Pour the mixture over the rice and mix well.

4 Spread 2–3 tablespoons of rice in an even layer over each nori sheet, leaving a 2cm/¾in gap at the top and bottom of the nori to allow you to roll it up. Press the rice down with the back of a teaspoon to make a compacted, firm base. Arrange 2 pieces each of the pepper and avocado in the centre of each sheet, then top with 2 teaspoons of the tofu mayonnaise.

5 Roll up each nori sheet – they should now look like Swiss rolls. Press gently to seal the edges of the rolls (the heat of the sushi rice should stick them together). If the ends do not stick together, wet the edges with a little water. Wrap the rolls tightly in cling film and chill in the fridge for 10 minutes.

6 Unwrap the rolls. Trim the ends with a knife and cut each one into 6 pieces. Divide into 4 equal portions and serve with soy sauce for dipping, and with wasabi paste and Japanese horseradish, if you like.

Nutritional analysis per serving: Calories 349.6kcal **Protein** 12.2g **Carbohydrates** 3.9g **Fat** 12.6g

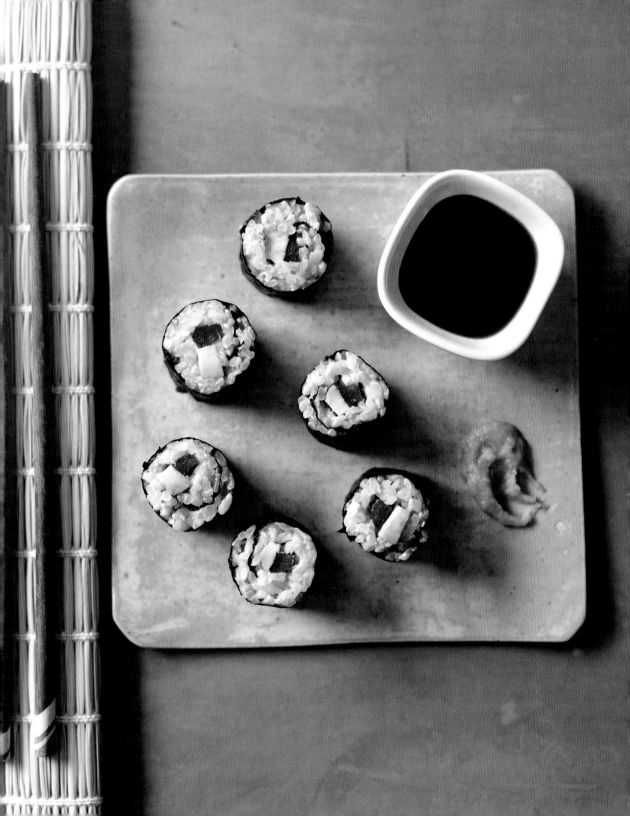

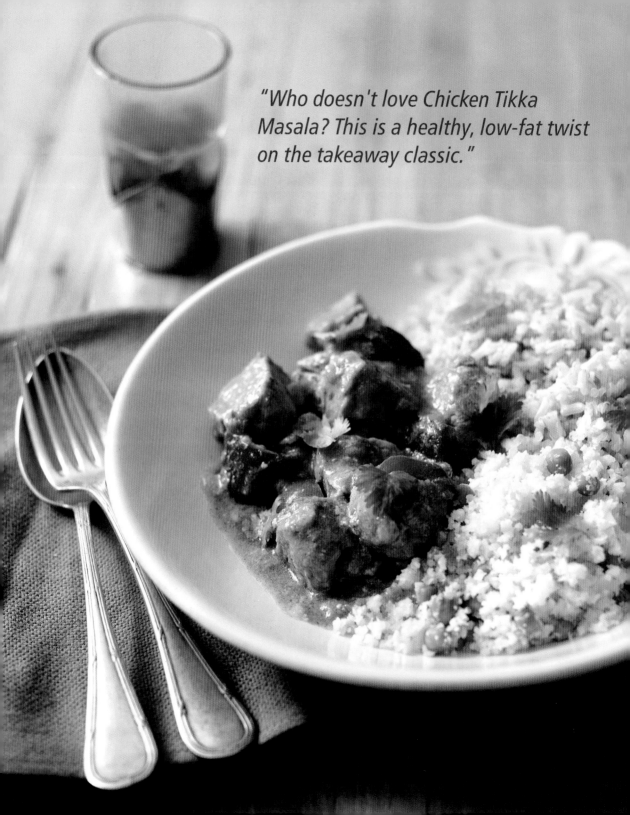

"Who doesn't love Chicken Tikka Masala? This is a healthy, low-fat twist on the takeaway classic."

Chicken Tikka Masala

MAKES: 4 servings
PREPARATION TIME: 15 minutes
COOKING TIME: 35 minutes

Rather than piling on the pounds with a takeaway, you can make the S Factor version of this classic curry instead. Vegetarians can replace the chicken with 500g/1lb 2oz silken tofu or Quorn.

150g/5½oz/scant ¾ cup brown rice
150g/5½oz/¾ cup quinoa
2 tsp coconut oil or extra virgin olive oil
1 small onion, finely chopped
2 garlic cloves
3cm/1¼in piece of root ginger, peeled and grated
a pinch of dried coriander
1 tsp garam masala
a pinch of paprika
a pinch of chilli powder
4 boneless, skinless chicken breasts, each about 200g/7oz, cut into bite-sized pieces or 500g/1lb 2oz silken tofu or Quorn, cut into bite-sized pieces
1 tsp tomato paste
1 green pepper, deseeded and cut into chunks
1 red pepper, deseeded and cut into chunks
juice of ½ lemon
1 cauliflower head, broken into florets
100g/3½oz/⅔ cup frozen peas, defrosted
100g/3½oz/heaped ⅓ cup reduced-fat Greek yogurt
fine sea salt and freshly ground black pepper
2 tbsp coriander leaves, to serve

1   Rinse the rice under cold running water for 1 minute, then drain. Put the rice and quinoa in a heavy-based saucepan and cover with water. Bring to the boil over a medium-high heat, then reduce the heat to low and simmer, covered, for 20 minutes until all the water has been absorbed. Remove the pan from the heat and leave to stand, covered, for 10 minutes.

2   Meanwhile, heat the coconut oil in a non-stick saucepan over a medium-high heat. Cook the onion and garlic for 4–5 minutes until the onion has softened. Add the ginger, spices and a pinch of salt, and cook, stirring, for 1–2 minutes. Add the chicken and cook for a further 2 minutes until browned all over, then stir in the tomato paste, peppers and a splash of lemon juice. Pour in 250ml/9fl oz/1 cup water and bring to the boil over a medium-high heat. Reduce the heat to low and simmer for 15–20 minutes until the chicken is cooked through and the sauce has thickened.

3   Ten minutes before the end of the cooking time, put the cauliflower in a food processor and process until it resembles coarse breadcrumbs. Transfer to a steamer, add the peas, then cover and steam for 2 minutes until heated through. Add the remaining lemon juice to the steamed cauliflower, then season with salt and pepper and stir. Remove the curry from the heat and stir in the yogurt. Divide the curry, rice and quinoa mix and cauliflower into 4 equal portions. Sprinkle with coriander and serve.

Nutritional analysis per serving: Calories 555kcal **Protein** 46g **Carbohydrates** 80g **Fat** 5g

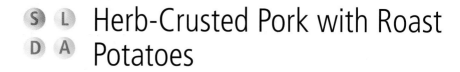

Herb-Crusted Pork with Roast Potatoes

MAKES: 4 servings
PREPARATION TIME: 20 minutes, plus 10 minutes resting
COOKING TIME: 1 hour

There are times when you want something really familiar. This pork dish is a low-fat take on a conventional roast, with an oat crust instead of fattening crackling. The roasties are still crisp and flavourful, but only have a fraction of their usual calories. It's an S Factor winner!

450g/1lb pork loin, skin and fat removed
60g/2¼oz/½ cup oatmeal
25g/1oz/¼ cup dried wholemeal breadcrumbs
1 tbsp chopped rosemary leaves
1 tbsp reduced-sugar apricot jam
500g/1lb 2oz roasting potatoes, such as Maris Piper
extra virgin olive oil cooking spray
1 tbsp chopped thyme leaves, plus extra sprigs to serve
coarse sea salt

1 Preheat the oven to 180°C/350°F/Gas 4. Put the pork in a roasting tin, then mix together the oatmeal, breadcrumbs and rosemary in a bowl. Brush the jam over the pork, making sure it is well coated. Spread the oatmeal mixture over the pork, pressing it down firmly to form a crust. Roast for 1 hour until cooked through. If the crust starts to burn, cover the pork with foil.

2 While the pork is roasting, peel the potatoes and cut each one into quarters. Put the potatoes in a large saucepan and cover with water. Bring to the boil over a medium-high heat, then reduce the heat to low and simmer for 10 minutes. Drain well, shaking the colander to rough up the edges of the potatoes – this will help them to crisp up in the oven.

3 Mist a baking tray with cooking spray, then spread the potatoes out in a single layer over the tray. Mist again with cooking spray, sprinkle with thyme and season with salt. Bake for 25–30 minutes, turning once, until golden.

4 Remove the pork from the oven, transfer to a plate and leave to rest for 10 minutes before slicing. Pour the cooking juices from the pork into a bowl and skim off any excess fat with a metal spoon. Sprinkle the pork and the potatoes with thyme sprigs, then divide into 4 equal portions. Spoon a little of the cooking juices over each portion and serve.

Nutritional analysis per serving: Calories 618kcal Protein 28.5g Carbohydrates 71g Fat 5.5g

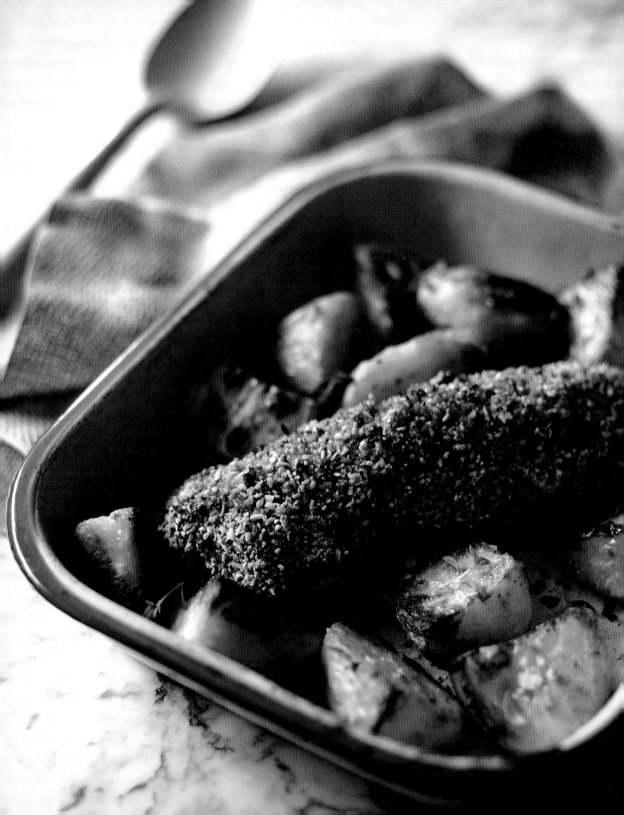

Fish, Chips & Mushy Peas

MAKES: 4 servings
PREPARATION TIME: 15 minutes
COOKING TIME: 40 minutes

This English classic is usually sky-high in fat, but this has a wholemeal crust and is baked in the oven. It's therefore lower in fat and with a high-fibre batter, so it's great for stabilizing blood sugar, energy and appetite.

extra virgin olive oil cooking spray
500g/1lb 2oz sweet potatoes, peeled and cut into thick chips
1 tsp fine sea salt, plus extra for seasoning the flour
3 slices of wholemeal bread, toasted, crusts removed and cut into small pieces
1 tbsp plain wholemeal flour
2 eggs, beaten
4 boneless, skinless white fish fillets such as pollock or hoki, each about 125g/4½oz
150g/5½oz/scant 1 cup frozen peas
2 tbsp chopped mint leaves
4 tbsp reduced-fat Greek yogurt
freshly ground black pepper

1 Preheat the oven to 200°C/400°F/Gas 6 and mist two baking trays with cooking spray. Put the sweet potatoes in a large saucepan and cover with water. Bring to the boil over a medium-high heat, then reduce the heat to low and simmer for 5–8 minutes. Drain well, shaking the colander to rough up the edges of the chips – this will help them to crisp up in the oven.

2 Spread the chips out in a single layer over one of the baking trays. Mist with cooking spray and sprinkle with the salt. Bake for 25–30 minutes, turning once, until golden.

3 Meanwhile, put the toasted bread in a food processor and process into coarse breadcrumbs. Put the breadcrumbs, flour and eggs in separate, shallow bowls. Season the flour with salt and pepper and mix.

4 Dip each fish fillet into the flour to coat well, shaking off any excess flour, then dip in the eggs and then in the breadcrumbs. Transfer the fish to the remaining baking tray and bake for 20 minutes until golden and crisp.

5 Ten minutes before the end of the cooking time, put the peas in a saucepan and cover with water. Bring to the boil over a medium-high heat and boil for 3–4 minutes until tender. Drain well, then return to the pan and mash coarsely with the back of a wooden spoon. Add the mint and yogurt and mix until combined. Divide the fish, chips and mushy peas into 4 equal portions and serve.

Nutritional analysis per serving: Calories 542kcal **Protein** 11.3g **Carbohydrates** 43.8g **Fat** 5.5g

Japanese Tuna Parcels with Wilted Greens

MAKES: 4 servings
PREPARATION TIME: 40 minutes
COOKING TIME: 20 minutes

If you want a great dinner party dish, this is it. The tuna steaks are cooked in parcels that your guests can unwrap at the table for a great "ta-da" moment! Plus, tuna is full of S Factor-friendly essential fats and proteins.

2 tsp sesame seeds
4 tuna steaks, each about 150g/5½oz, cut into bite-sized pieces or 600g/1lb 5oz tofu cut into bite-sized pieces
3cm/1¼in piece of root ginger, peeled and cut into slices with a vegetable peeler
2 celery sticks, sliced
4 spring onions, thinly sliced
¼ tsp dashi stock granules
3 tbsp mirin or dry sherry
2 tbsp tamari soy sauce
300g/10½oz cooked quinoa or 4 small baked potatoes, to serve

FOR THE GREENS:

2 tbsp soy sauce
a splash of white rice vinegar
3cm/1¼in piece of root ginger, peeled and grated
a squeeze of orange juice
1 tsp tahini
100g/3½oz baby spinach

1 Preheat the oven to 230°C/450°F/Gas 8 and cut four rectangles of baking parchment, each one large enough to enclose a tuna steak. Heat a non-stick frying pan over a medium heat. Dry-fry the sesame seeds for 1 minute, stirring occasionally, until golden and lightly toasted. Watch carefully so they do not burn. Remove from the heat and leave to one side.

2 Wash the tuna steaks under cold running water and pat dry with kitchen paper. Place one tuna steak in the centre of each parchment rectangle and top each one with one-quarter of the ginger, celery and spring onions. Leave to one side.

3 Put the dashi, mirin and tamari in a saucepan. Heat over a low heat, stirring, until the dashi has completely dissolved.

4 Sprinkle one-quarter of the dashi mixture and toasted sesame seeds over the top of each tuna steak. Gather up the edges of the parchment and tie with kitchen string to make 4 parcels. Bake for 12 minutes until the tuna steaks are opaque and cooked through.

5 Meanwhile, heat a wok over a medium heat. Add all of the ingredients for the greens except the spinach and stir until combined. Gradually add the spinach to the wok and toss for 2 minutes until wilted and well coated. Divide the greens into 4 equal portions and add a tuna parcel to each plate. Serve with cooked quinoa or small baked potatoes.

Nutritional analysis per serving: Calories 192kcal **Protein** 59g **Carbohydrates** 1.5g **Fat** 3.4g

Ⓢ Ⓛ Mini Mango & Passion Fruit Ⓓ Ⓐ Pavlovas

MAKES: 4 servings
PREPARATION TIME: 15 minutes, plus cooling
COOKING TIME: 20 minutes

You have to make meringues with sugar (I've tried with natural sweetener and they went droopy), but there's plenty of protein from the egg whites to offset that. Mango is high in resistant starch which speeds up metabolism and reduces appetite – so this recipe is especially useful if you have issues with leptin.

2 egg whites
½ tsp cornflour
½ tsp raspberry vinegar or white wine vinegar
90g/3¼oz/½ cup light muscovado sugar
150g/5½oz/scant ⅔ cup reduced-fat fromage frais
2 tsp agave syrup
1 mango, peeled and sliced
1 passion fruit, halved, to serve
25g/1oz pistachios, chopped, to serve

1 Preheat the oven to 160°C/315°F/Gas 2–3 and line a baking sheet with baking parchment. Whisk the egg whites in a clean bowl until they form stiff peaks. Whisk in the cornflour and vinegar, then gradually add the sugar, whisking after each addition, until the mixture is stiff and glossy.

2 Spoon one-quarter of the mixure onto the baking sheet, then shape into a circle and flatten the top slightly with the back of a metal spoon. Repeat with the remaining mixture to make 4 circles, spacing them apart. Bake for 20 minutes until firm on the outside but soft in the centre. Remove from the oven and leave to cool.

3 Put the fromage frais and agave syrup in a bowl and mix until combined. Top each pavlova with one-quarter of the mango and 2 tablespoons of the fromage frais mixture. Spoon the flesh from the passion fruit evenly over the top of each pavlova, sprinkle with pistachios and serve.

Nutritional analysis per serving: Calories 221kcal **Protein** 6.9g **Carbohydrates** 43g **Fat** 3.6g

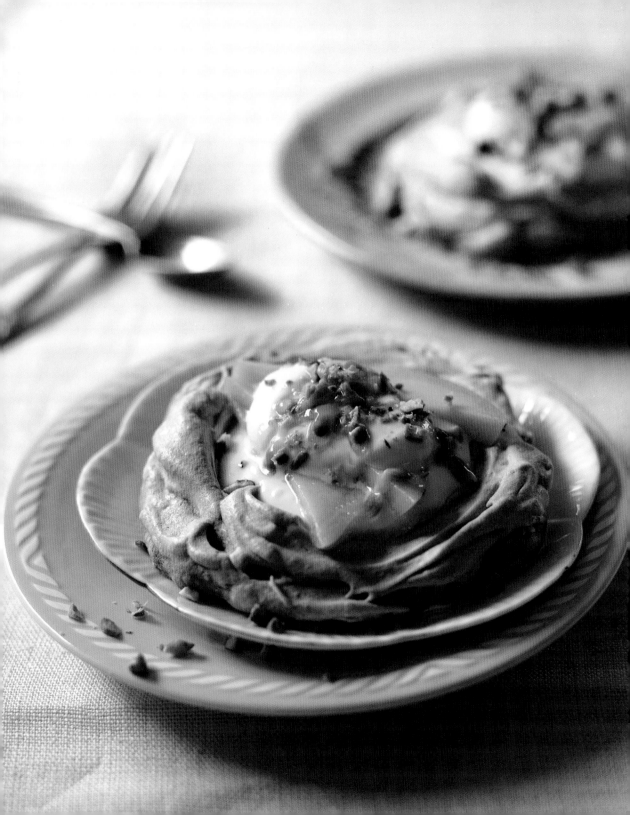

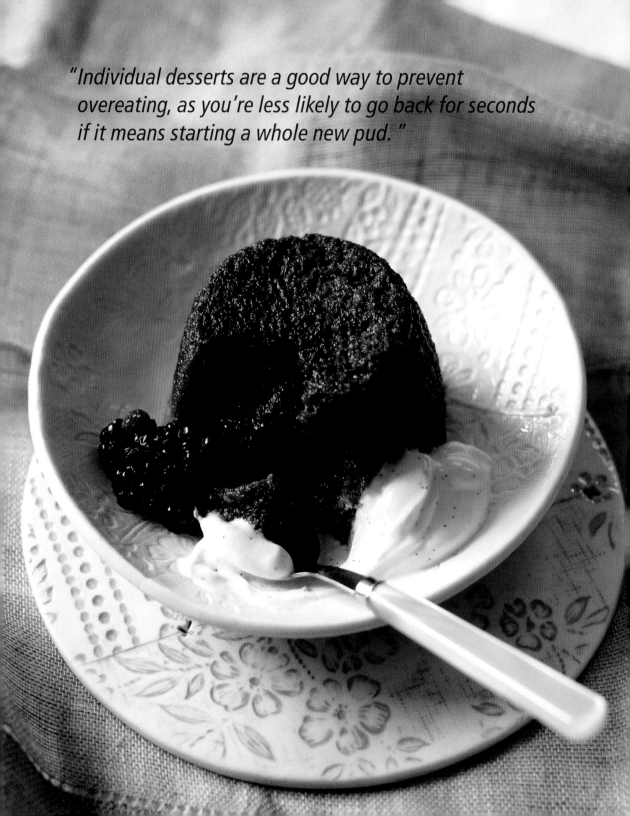

"Individual desserts are a good way to prevent overeating, as you're less likely to go back for seconds if it means starting a whole new pud."

Baby Summer Puddings

MAKES: 6 servings
PREPARATION TIME: 15 minutes,
plus cooling and 4 hours chilling
COOKING TIME: 15 minutes

extra virgin olive oil cooking spray
100g/3½oz/½ cup stevia-based natural
   sweetener or xylitol
zest of ½ lemon
400g/14oz summer berries such as red
   currants, raspberries and blackberries
24 thin slices of wholemeal bread,
   crusts removed
½ vanilla pod, seeds scraped out or
   2 drops of vanilla extract
100g/3½oz/heaped ⅓ cup reduced-fat
   crème fraîche

1 Mist six 175ml/5½fl oz/⅔-cup pudding basins or teacups with cooking spray and line with cling flim, leaving enough of an overhang to enclose the puddings. Put the natural sweetener, lemon zest and 75ml/2¼fl oz/generous ¼ cup water in a saucepan. Heat over a low heat, stirring, until the natural sweetener has dissolved and the mixture is syrupy. Increase the heat to medium-low and simmer for 5 minutes until thickened. Remove the pan from the heat and leave to cool a little.

2 Pour half of the syrup into a blender. Add 50g/1¾oz of the berries and purée until smooth. Using the back of a metal spoon, press the mixture through a sieve into a clean bowl. Discard the seeds.

3 Add the remaining berries to the syrup in the saucepan. Heat over a low heat and simmer for 1–2 minutes until the berries begin to soften. Add the puréed syrup and berry mixture and stir until combined. Strain the juices into one bowl and pour the softened berries into another, then leave to cool completely.

4 Take 6 slices of bread and, using the base of one of the pudding basins as a template, cut out 6 circles. Discard the leftover edges. Dip the bread circles and remaining slices into the juices until well coated but not soaked, then transfer to a plate. Reserve and chill any remaining juices.

5 Line the bottom and sides of each basin with 3 slices of soaked bread, then evenly spoon the softened berries into each one. Top each pudding with a soaked circle of bread to enclose the filling, then fold the cling film over the tops to seal. Put a ramekin on top of each pudding and weight them down with bags of dried beans or tins of food. Chill in the fridge for 4 hours until set.

6 Mix together the vanilla seeds and crème fraîche in a bowl. Turn the puddings out of the basins and drizzle the reserved juices over the top. Serve each pudding with one-quarter of the crème fraîche.

Nutritional analysis per serving: Calories 346kcal **Protein** 4.7g **Carbohydrates** 22g **Fat** 3.6g

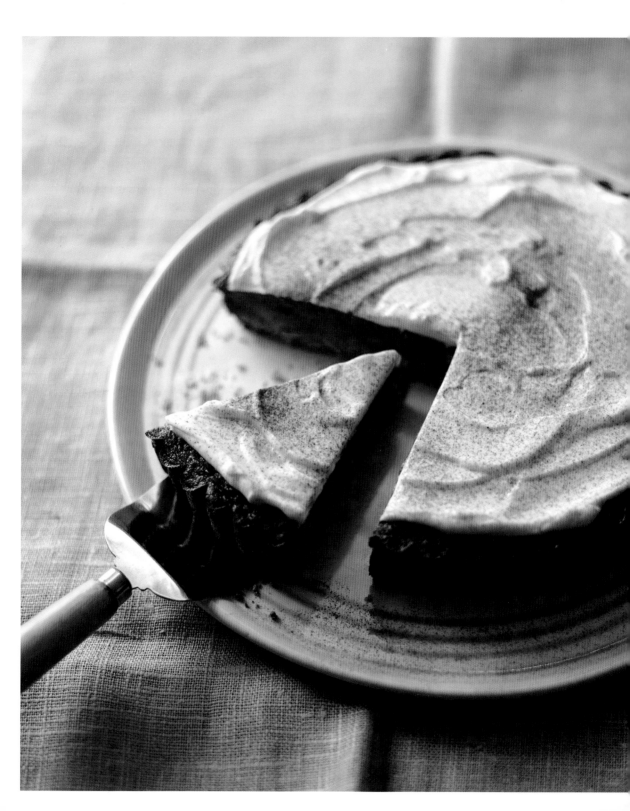

American-Style Pumpkin Pie

MAKES: 8 servings
PREPARATION TIME: 15 minutes,
plus 20 minutes chilling, and cooling
COOKING TIME: 1 hour

Americans often use pumpkin in sweet pies. Pumpkin has the advantage for S Factor dieters of being high in resistant starch which helps balance leptin levels. It's also low GI, so it keeps energy, mood and cravings under control.

FOR THE PASTRY:
extra virgin olive oil cooking spray
100g/3½oz/⅔ cup plain wholemeal
    flour
90g/3¼oz/scant 1 cup ground almonds
50g/1¾oz/heaped ¼ cup stevia-based
    natural sweetener or xylitol
100g/3½oz chilled butter, diced
½ egg yolk

FOR THE FILLING:
500g/1lb 2oz pumpkin, peeled,
    deseeded and cut into chunks
3 eggs, beaten
3 tbsp stevia-based natural sweetener
    or xylitol
1½ tsp ground cinnamon, plus extra
    to serve
1 tsp ground ginger
a pinch of ground allspice
a pinch of ground cloves
a pinch of ground cardamom
a pinch of fine sea salt
4 tbsp reduced-fat Greek yogurt

1   Mist a loose-based, 20cm/8in pie dish with cooking spray. Put all of the ingredients for the pastry, except the egg yolk, in a food processor and pulse until the mixture resembles coarse breadcrumbs. Add the egg yolk and pulse again to form a soft dough.

2   Press the dough into the bottom (not the sides) of the pie dish and chill in the freezer for 20 minutes. Preheat the oven to 190°C/375°F/Gas 5. Remove the pie dish from the freezer and blind bake for 15 minutes until golden.

3   Meanwhile, make the filling. Put the pumpkin in a steamer, or in a colander over a pan with about 5cm/2in water and bring to the boil. Cover and steam for 10–15 minutes until softened. Transfer to a sieve and press down with the back of a wooden spoon to remove as much water as possible, discarding the water. Put the pumpkin in a bowl and mash thoroughly until smooth. Leave to cool completely.

4   In large bowl, beat together the eggs and natural sweetener. Add the mashed pumpkin, spices and salt and stir until well combined.

5   Remove the pie dish from the oven and pour the filling over the pastry. Bake for 10 minutes, then turn the oven down to 180°C/350°F/Gas 4 and bake for a further 30 minutes until the filling has set and a skewer inserted in the centre comes out clean.

6   Remove the pie from the oven and leave in the tin to cool completely. Turn out of the tin and transfer to a plate. Spread the yogurt in an even layer over the top of the pie. Dust with cinnamon, cut the pie into 8 equal slices and serve.

Nutritional analysis per serving: Calories 255kcal **Protein** 5.2g **Carbohydrates** 11g **Fat** 18.6g

Chocolate & Avocado Truffles

MAKES: 6 servings (18 truffles)
PREPARATION TIME: 15 minutes,
plus at least 1 hour chilling

These are my all-time favourite chocolates and are a lovely healthy treat if you don't go mad with them. The avocado gives a silky texture in place of cream. You don't taste it in the finished truffles and, don't worry, they don't turn out green either, because of the cocoa.

2 avocados, peeled, pitted and chopped
60g/2¼oz coconut butter
50ml/1½fl oz/3 tbsp agave syrup
60g/2¼oz/½ cup cocoa powder, sifted,
    plus extra for coating and dusting

1 Put all of the ingredients in a food processor and process until smooth.

2 Sprinkle 3 tablespoons of cocoa powder into a shallow bowl. Dust your hands with a little more cocoa powder and divide the truffle mixture into 18 equal pieces. Shape each one into a ball, then roll in the cocoa powder until completely coated, shaking off any excess.

3 Transfer to a plate and chill in the fridge for 1–2 hours until set. Divide into 6 equal portions and serve.

Nutritional analysis per serving: **Calories** 242kcal **Protein** 3.2g **Carbohydrates** 8.2g **Fat** 61.5g

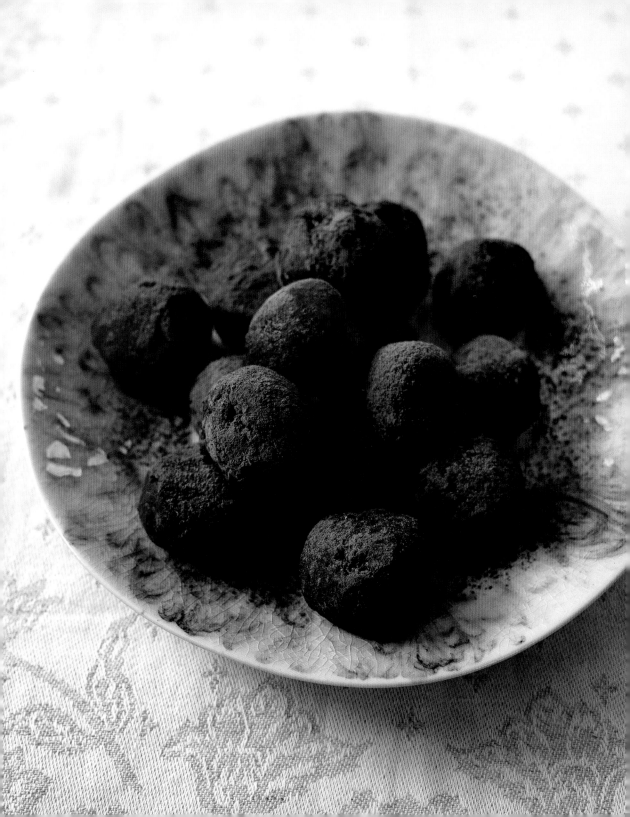

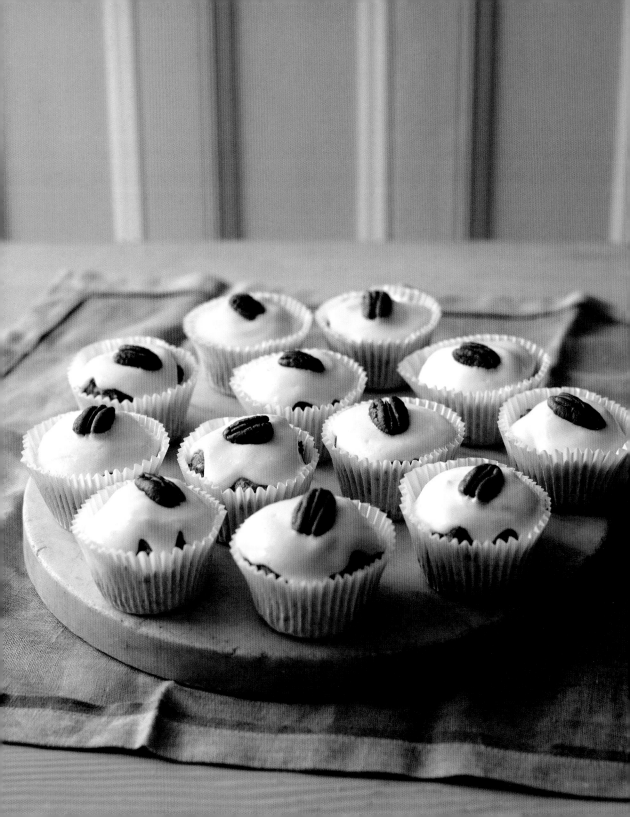

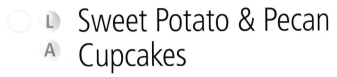

Sweet Potato & Pecan Cupcakes

MAKES: 12 servings (12 cupcakes)
PREPARATION TIME: 20 minutes, plus cooling
COOKING TIME: 50 minutes

These are a good alternative to carrot cakes. Sweet potatoes have a similar natural sweetness but are higher in resistant starch, so are better at creating a feeling of fullness, which is important for the leptin-deprived.

225g/8oz sweet potatoes, cut into chunks
125g/4½oz/½ cup reduced-fat Greek yogurt
1 egg, beaten
1 tsp vanilla extract
80g/2¾oz/scant ⅔ cup white self-raising flour
100g/3½oz/⅔ cup plain wholemeal flour
1 tsp baking powder
½ tsp ground cinnamon
a pinch of ground ginger
a pinch of ground allspice
a pinch of salt
115g/4oz/½ cup + 1 tbsp stevia-based natural sweetener or xylitol
150g/5½oz/1½ cups pecan nuts, chopped, plus 12 pecan halves to decorate

FOR THE FROSTING:
250g/9oz/1 cup reduced-fat cream cheese
110g/3¾oz/heaped ½ cup stevia-based natural sweetener or xylitol

1 Preheat the oven to 180°C/350°F/Gas 4 and arrange 12 paper cupcake cases in a 12-hole bun tin. Put the sweet potatoes in a large saucepan and cover with water. Bring to the boil over a medium-high heat, then reduce the heat to low and simmer for 20–25 minutes until completely soft. Drain well and leave to cool a little. Transfer to a large bowl and mash thoroughly until smooth.

2 Add the yogurt, egg and vanilla extract to the sweet potatoes and mix well. Sift the flours, baking powder, spices and salt into another bowl, then stir in the natural sweetener. Gradually fold the flour mixture into the sweet potato mixture, but take care not to overmix. Fold in the chopped pecans and divide the mixture evenly into the cupcake cases.

3 Bake for 20–25 minutes until firm to the touch and a skewer inserted in the centre comes out clean. Remove from the oven and leave to cool in the tin for 5 minutes, then transfer to a wire rack and leave to cool completely.

4 To make the frosting, beat together the cream cheese and natural sweetener in a bowl. Spread 2 teaspoons of the frosting over each cupcake, top with a pecan half and serve.

Nutritional analysis per serving: Calories 198kcal **Protein** 4g **Carbohydrates** 14.8g **Fat** 12.5g

High-Protein Cranberry Brownies

S ○
D ○

These protein-rich brownies are brilliant for balancing serotonin and dopamine levels. They have a gorgeous sweet, chocolatey taste, plus the cranberries add a great sharpness. The perfect bedtime snack.

MAKES: 6 servings (12 brownies)
PREPARATION TIME: 10 minutes, plus cooling
COOKING TIME: 25 minutes

extra virgin olive oil cooking spray
75g/2½oz/scant ⅔ cup self-raising flour
40g/1½oz/⅓ cup cocoa powder
175g/6oz/¾ cup + 2 tbsp stevia-based natural sweetener or xylitol
25g/1oz walnuts, chopped
100g/3½oz/heaped ⅓ cup reduced-fat vanilla yogurt
3 eggs, beaten
1 tsp vanilla extract
1½ tsp extra virgin olive oil
25g/1oz cranberries

1 Preheat the oven to 180°C/350°F/Gas 4 and mist a 18 x 18cm/7 x 7in baking tin with cooking spray. Sift the flour and cocoa powder into a mixing bowl, then add the natural sweetener and walnuts and mix well. In another bowl, beat together the yogurt, eggs, vanilla extract and olive oil. Gradually add the egg mixture to the flour mixture and beat until well combined, but take care not to overmix. Carefully fold in the cranberries with a metal spoon.

2 Spoon the mixture into the baking tin and smooth the surface with the back of a metal spoon. Bake for 25 minutes until firm to the touch and a skewer inserted in the centre comes out clean.

3 Remove from the oven and cut into 12 equal squares. Transfer to a wire rack and leave to cool completely, then serve.

Nutritional analysis per serving: Calories 163.5kcal **Protein** 5g **Carbohydrates** 12.9g **Fat** 10.1g

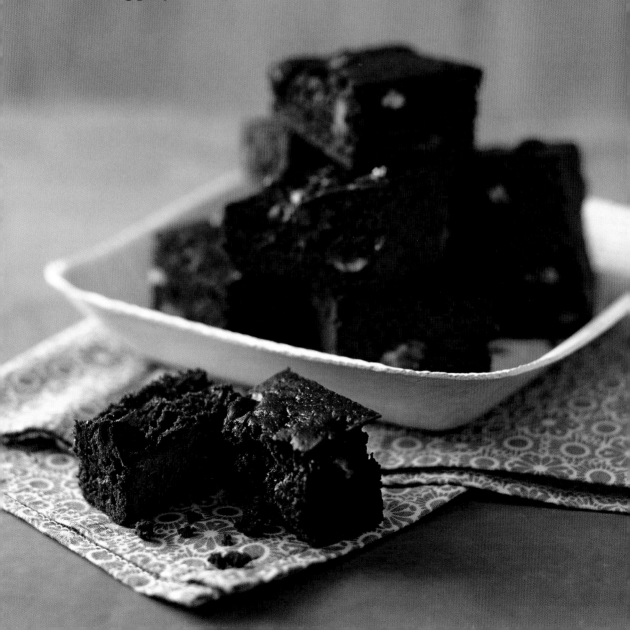

"Brownies can't really be good for you, can they?
Well, if they're made of protein-packed yogurt and
eggs, yes they can!"

Chocolate-Dipped Pretzels

MAKES: 4 servings
PREPARATION TIME: 10 minutes, plus 10 minutes chilling
COOKING TIME: 5 minutes

Chocolate is a fantastic way to balance serotonin, but there's no getting round it – it's very high in calories. To keep your weight under control then, you need to find ways to make a little chocolate go a long way. These pretzels are chocolatey enough to satisfy a choccy craving, but won't pile on the pounds.

75g/2½oz dark chocolate, 70% cocoa solids, broken into squares
50g/1¾oz mini salted pretzels

1 Line a cooling rack with baking parchment. Put the chocolate in a heatproof bowl and rest it over a saucepan of gently simmering water, making sure the bottom of the bowl does not touch the water. Heat, stirring occasionally, until the chocolate has melted. Alternatively, melt the chocolate in a glass bowl in the microwave in 10-second spurts – watch carefully to make sure it does not burn.

2 Dip one side of each pretzel into the melted chocolate and transfer to the cooling rack. Leave to cool a little then transfer to a plate and chill in the fridge for 10 minutes. Divide into 4 equal portions and serve.

Nutritional analysis per serving: Calories 140kcal **Protein** 1.3g **Carbohydrates** 18.3g **Fat** 6.3g

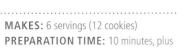

Almond Butter Cookies

MAKES: 6 servings (12 cookies)
PREPARATION TIME: 10 minutes, plus cooling and 10 minutes chilling
COOKING TIME: 10 minutes

Peanut butter cookies are a common favourite, but peanuts, which are a ground nut, have less nutritional value than tree nuts such as walnuts, Brazils and almonds. You can buy almond butter in a jar just like peanut butter. Whey powder, which you can buy from health food stores, replaces flour to push up the protein content.

50g/1¾oz softened butter
30g/1oz almond butter
2 tbsp agave syrup
100g/3½oz/scant ⅔ cup brown rice flour
100g/3½oz chocolate whey powder
½ tsp baking powder
20g/¾oz flaked almonds
25g/1oz white chocolate, roughly chopped

1 Preheat the oven to 180°C/350°F/Gas 4 and line a baking sheet with baking parchment. Put the butters and agave syrup in a bowl and beat until light and fluffy. Add the rice flour, whey powder and baking powder. Beat slowly with a wooden spoon until just combined, but take care not to overmix.

2 Put the almonds in a shallow bowl. Using your hands, divide the cookie mixture into 12 equal pieces and shape each one into a ball. Roll the balls of cookie dough in the almonds, then transfer to the baking sheet, spacing them well apart. Flatten the tops slightly with a spatula and bake for 8–10 minutes until golden. Remove from the oven and leave to cool completely.

3 Line a cooling rack with baking parchment. Put the chocolate in a heatproof bowl and rest it over a saucepan of gently simmering water, making sure the bottom of the bowl does not touch the water. Heat, stirring occasionally, until the chocolate has melted. Alternatively, melt the chocolate in a glass bowl in the microwave in 10-second spurts – watch carefully to make sure it does not burn. Drizzle the chocolate evenly over the cookies and transfer to the cooling rack. Leave to cool a little until the chocolate has set, then transfer to a plate and chill in the fridge for 10 minutes. Divide into 6 equal portions and serve.

Nutritional analysis per serving: Calories 153kcal **Protein** 18g **Carbohydrates** 14.5g **Fat** 13.8g

The S Factor Diet – Final Thought

Anyone who used to watch *The Jerry Springer Show* will be familiar with the point at the end of the programme when Jerry gave us his homespun "Final Thought". I wanted to end this book with my own final thought, something that would encourage and inspire you.

I certainly would have liked someone in my corner over the years I spent battling food. Food obsession can be very isolating. The dialogue in your head about what you've eaten today, what you shouldn't have eaten today, and what you're not going to eat tomorrow can be all-consuming – especially if you keep it a secret from others.

I see lots of intelligent, successful people at my clinic who are in control of every area of their lives, except their eating habits. They keep their food obsession a secret out of embarrassment and shame. They feel powerless. I'll tell you what I tell them: "You are not powerless". Your power is just buried under a hormonal tsunami. Get your S Factor hormones working properly and you can regain your balance in every sense.

You'll have to work at it, but the rewards come surprisingly quickly. Once your S Factor hormones are balanced, it's amazing how the cravings recede. Take it one meal at a time and just do your best. You don't have to be perfect. Good enough is good enough.

One problem many of my clients have is other people, as they come under pressure to eat foods that aren't on their S Factor plan. My answer to this is to be polite, but firm. There is a useful phrase to remember here: "No" is a complete sentence. You don't have to explain or justify why you don't want to eat that slice of pizza or chocolate cake. Just say, "no, thank you" and leave it at that.

The S Factor diet doesn't come with a magic wand. Completing the programme doesn't mean you'll never want chocolate again. Our default settings are stubborn. When I take on too much, I very quickly spin into a vortex of stress – I stop looking after myself and I stop eating properly. Fortunately, I can now pull myself out of these whirlwinds pretty quickly. The good thing about having a bit of a blip is that when you go back to eating properly, you'll discover all over again how much better you feel on the wagon than off it.

You will inevitably falter from time to time. But, as the saying goes, it's a marathon not a sprint. If you do have a bad day, get right back on track the day after. The fantastic thing about your weight is that it's one of the few things in life which will always give you a second chance, third chance, fourth chance…. Mess up in your job and you might get sacked, do something terrible to your partner and your relationship might be over. But when you eat a whole packet of biscuits, you can get up the next day with a clean slate and start again. It's never too late to eat properly, to invest in yourself and to have the body you'd like to have.

Jerry used to sign off by saying, "Take care of yourselves and each other". I'll sign off by saying, "Be kind to your body – and yourself".

Index